Social Inclusion of People with Mental Illness

People with serious mental illness no longer spend years of their lives in psychiatric institutions. In developed countries, there has been a major shift in the focus of care from hospitals into the community. However, whilst it means those with mental illness are not confined, it does not guarantee they will be fully integrated into their communities. The barriers to full citizenship are partly due to the disabilities produced by their illnesses and partly by stigmatising and discriminatory attitudes of the public. This book analyses the causes of these barriers and suggests ways of dismantling them. The book is constructed in two parts, the first relates to social inclusion and the second to occupational inclusion. Throughout, the text is annotated with quotes from consumers, to illustrate their experience of the issues discussed. The innovations outlined are described in sufficient detail for the reader to implement them in their own practice.

Julian Leff is Emeritus Professor at the Institute of Psychiatry and Royal Free and University College Medical School, London.

Richard Warner is Professor of Psychiatry and Adjunct Professor of Anthropology at the University of Colorado, and Director of Colorado Recovery in Boulder, a program providing intensive community-based care for people with schizophrenia and related disorders.

Social Inclusion of People with Mental Illness

Julian Leff

Richard Warner

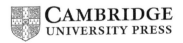

CAMBRIDGE
UNIVERSITY PRESS

CAMBRIDGE UNIVERSITY PRESS
Cambridge, New York, Melbourne, Madrid, Cape Town, Singapore, São Paulo

CAMBRIDGE UNIVERSITY PRESS
The Edinburgh Building, Cambridge CB2 2RU, UK
Published in the United States of America by Cambridge University Press, New York

www.cambridge.org
Information on this title: www.cambridge.org/9780521615365

First published 2006

Printed in the United Kingdom at the University Press, Cambridge

A catalogue record for this publication is available from the British Library

Library of Congress Cataloguing in Publication data
Leff, Julian P.
     The social inclusion of people with mental illness/Julian Leff,
Richard Warner.
          p.   cm.
     Includes bibliographical references and index.
     ISBN-13: 978-0-521-61536-5 (paperback)
     ISBN-10: 0-521-61536-4 (paperback)
     1. Mental illness.   2. Mental illness – Social aspects.   I. Warner,
Richard, 1943– .   II. Title.
     [DNLM: 1. Mental Disorders.   2. Socioeconomic Factors.   3. Social
Isolation – psychology.   WM 31 L493s 2006]
     RC454 . L374 2006
     362.196'89dc22   2006008745

ISBN-13 978-0-521-61536-5 paperback
ISBN-10 0-521-61536-4 paperback

Contents

Preface

This is a tale of two systems – the systems of care for people with mental illness in Britain and the USA. Although both the authors are British-trained, one (JL) has practised social and community psychiatry in the UK and the other (RW) in the USA. We have both, however, had ample opportunity to visit the service systems in these two countries and in many others around the world. This exposure to different systems of care has allowed us to present quite a broad range of experiences and models to the reader, but, here and there, it may have introduced a note of confusion.

In Britain, for example, the current term for someone who has experienced an episode of mental illness and has received mental health services is a 'service-user' or 'user'. In the USA, the term is 'consumer'. After struggling with this for a while, we gave up and left you, the reader, to sort it out. Just remember: service-user = user = consumer.

More complicated is the fact that the systems in which we have worked in Britain and the USA developed quite differently after the Second World War, and so the models of treatment and rehabilitation that we have helped to develop were designed to respond to different problems. This is an important lesson in itself. The treatment approaches and models that we describe in this book did not happen in a vacuum – they are responses to specific conditions. An anti-stigma programme in Philadelphia, for example, may need to focus on the police force, because that is the first point of contact for many acutely disturbed people with mental illness in that city. In Glasgow, the same effort might best be expended on family doctors. Similarly, service managers will decide what programme innovation is needed most urgently based on what is the biggest perceived problem, be it the 'revolving-door patient' who relapses several times a year and is repeatedly admitted to hospital, or the person whose symptoms of mental illness are in good remission but whose life is empty and meaningless. Because the context is so important, we will describe here some of the differences between the mental health treatment systems in Britain and the USA in recent decades, because these differences influenced the direction that we both took in our work.

Something of a revolution in the treatment of people with serious mental illness was taking place in post-war northern Europe, even before antipsychotic drugs were introduced in 1954 – a revolution that went unnoticed in the USA until it was well under way. British psychiatrists transformed the psychiatric hospitals by abolishing the use of restraints and seclusion, mixing the genders, unlocking the doors and establishing power-sharing therapeutic communities in which staff and patients shared in decision-making about the hospital environment and its management. Group homes were developed for long-hospitalised patients to live in the community. In so doing, northern European psychiatrists stole a march on the rest of the world in developing treatment environments that fostered recovery from psychosis and an early return to community living. This progress slowed down for a while in Britain after 1970, when the Seebohm Report led to a statutory division between funding for community support and treatment services.

While dramatic changes were taking place in post-war northern Europe, most of the US asylums remained backward and repressive. This provided the moral and philosophical basis for a massive deinstitutionalisation movement that was launched in the USA in the late 1950s. The movement was politically driven, however, by the introduction of the Medicaid health insurance programme, which divided the cost of community care for people with mental illness 50/50 between the state and federal governments, in contrast to state hospital care, which continued to rest entirely on the shoulders of the state government. Most of the discharged state hospital patients ended up in substandard conditions in boarding homes and nursing homes, a situation that was soon to be recognised as a national scandal. The development of a network of community mental health centres after 1965, which often focused efforts on people with lesser disorders, did little initially to help the plight of these ex-hospital patients.

So, in the 1970s, while there were still many patients in long-term hospital care in Britain, in the USA there were huge numbers of 'revolving-door patients' with very little in the way of community care or supportive services. The US services tackled their primary challenge by developing assertive community treatment services to prevent relapse and hospital admission. Many British services, on the other hand, were still dealing with patients who had been in hospital for decades and were suffering the consequences – symptoms such as agitation, passivity, pacing and incontinence. The best British services developed residential treatment settings to move long-hospitalised patients into more domestic living environments in the community. When pressure mounted in the 1980s to close more British asylums, many of the treatment services expanded their network of residential settings and developed home services provided by community nurses. As the hospital closures advanced, often these measures were inadequate to meet the demands created by the new young clients with serious mental illnesses. Many acute hospitals and community treatment teams found themselves overstretched. British services began to examine US and Australian models that had been developed in order to address these problems, especially assertive community treatment and crisis intervention.

At the time of writing, the two systems are more similar than they have been for decades. Both systems have developed methods to prevent relapse and to get along with few acute psychiatric hospital beds. Both are now grappling with the issues that we deal with in this book. How do we help people with psychosis who are living in the community become *citizens* of that community? How do we help them find valued social roles and to escape poverty, victimisation and, sometimes, prison incarceration? How do we help the community to see these people as fully entitled, fully human community members? Recovery from mental illness is about more than just getting rid of the symptoms and staying out of hospital. It is about regaining a sense of identity, belonging and meaning in life.

To illustrate this process of recovery, we collaborated with two researchers from Brisbane, Vaidyanathan Kalyanasundaram and Barbara Tooth, who are experienced in interviewing people with serious mental illness about aspects of their lives that allowed them to achieve mastery of their mental illnesses. With another interviewer, who has mental illness herself, they interviewed 20 people in Boulder, Colorado, all of whom had overcome the obstacles presented by psychotic illness to lead full and productive lives. The comments of these consumers on coping strategies, work, stigma, speaking out, obstacles and optimism are introduced in the relevant sections throughout this book. We are most grateful for their contributions.

Introduction: barriers to social and occupational integration

The focus in this book is on people with serious mental illnesses, particularly psychoses, schizophrenia and manic-depressive illness (termed bipolar illness in the USA). Although less serious psychiatric conditions such as depression may also lead to social and occupational exclusion, the barriers are not as formidable or as extensive as with the psychotic illnesses. Perhaps this is because the latter often produce symptoms with which the person in the street cannot empathise. One of us (JL) was sharing the platform at a public meeting with Lewis Wolpert, who has written and spoken extensively about the severe depressive illness he suffered in the past and from which he has fully recovered. He told the audience that it took a great effort for him to overcome his reluctance to expose his experience to the public because of the considerable stigma accorded to depression. JL followed this confession by relating that when patients in his care who suffer from schizophrenia ask him how to explain the gaps in their work record to a potential employer, he advises them to say that they have been depressed.

1.1 Disabilities produced by the illness

The barriers are partly attributable to the effects of the illness and its management by professionals and partly to the reaction of the public. Both schizophrenia and manic-depressive illness commonly lead to delusions – false beliefs about the world – and hallucinations – seeing or hearing things that others do not experience. These symptoms can dominate patients' lives and interfere with their ability to interact with others, to attend to tasks and to think clearly.

Schizophrenia can also produce apathy, lack of interest, lack of motivation and a reluctance to engage with other people. These symptoms make it very difficult for the patient to undertake the search for a job, let alone to negotiate an interview, meet the demands of a job or form relationships with workmates. The symptoms also inhibit the activity of making and keeping friends. These negative symptoms, as they are termed, are much commoner in schizophrenia than in manic-depressive illness, but they do appear in the depressed phase of the latter condition. Both positive and negative symptoms can respond to treatment, but all treatments have unwanted side effects.

1.2 Disabilities produced by professional care

The massive development of asylums in the UK in the nineteenth century was initiated as a solution to scandalous conditions in the private 'madhouses'. They became the centres of psychiatric care throughout the developed world and were exported to developing countries by the colonial powers. Although asylums were designed, with the best of intentions, to provide recreational spaces and the free circulation of air, they rapidly became overcrowded and understaffed. Constructed to house several hundred patients, many of them reached a peak of over two thousand. Those patients who could not be conscripted into a labour force to service and maintain the asylum were consigned to 'back wards', where they suffered neglect and inactivity. The lack of any occupation increased the severity of the apathy and inertia produced by their illnesses.

This was not the only deleterious effect of the institutions. They also came to represent to the public places into which disturbed patients disappeared, never to emerge again. Thus, they became readily identifiable icons of the stigma of mental illness. The introduction in the 1950s of effective medication to treat psychiatric disorders hastened the discharge of patients into the community, which had begun a few years earlier in the late 1940s. Unfortunately, these valuable drugs had side effects that produced conspicuous abnormalities of movement and behaviour. The mildest effects were shaking of the hands and a tendency to shuffle when walking, but patients could also suffer from major spasms of the head, neck and tongue, and even difficulties in breathing evenly and in speaking. Some patients were left with a constant flow of saliva, which dribbled from their mouths. These peculiarities marked the patients out as different from their healthy neighbours and compounded the stigma of their illnesses.

1.3 Attitudes of the public

Throughout the world, people with serious mental illnesses are viewed differently from those with physical illnesses. This is attributable partly to a perceived link with violence, which will be discussed below, and partly to difficulties in sharing and understanding the abnormal experiences that are induced by schizophrenia and manic-depressive illness. Members of the public wish to distance themselves from people with such illnesses, as shown by their reluctance to work with them, marry them, live close to them, and have them as friends. In developed countries, a small minority of neighbours resist the establishment of sheltered housing in their streets and become very vocal in their resistance, sometimes defeating the efforts of service providers to sway the public towards acceptance.

Stigmatising attitudes vary with age and sex, older people being more prejudiced than younger people, and women more than men. Women with children are particularly fearful of people with mental illness, believing that their young ones are at risk of being harmed. Rejection by the public of people with psychiatric disorders leads to social isolation of the patients and results in their segregation with other people with similar mental health problems. It becomes very difficult for an individual to break out of this social ghetto.

1.4 Influence of the media

The media are very influential in the formation of public attitudes, and journalists working in newspapers and television have the power either to dispel or to reinforce misconceptions about mental illnesses. Journalists might be expected to be better informed than the general public about mental illness, but unfortunately this is rarely the case. Headlines and news stories tend to dramatise the rare occasions when a member of the public is harmed or killed by a person suffering from a mental illness. The language used is often pejorative, with slang terms such as 'weirdo' and 'nutcase'. The constant linking of mental illness with violence creates or strengthens an already existing stereotype.

Stigma in the community

They used to call me names. People that I met on the streets. They called me 'wing-nut' and stuff like that because of my mental illness. That kind of hurt me. It doesn't happen so much now.

Local newspapers can mount campaigns against the setting up of sheltered homes in a neighbourhood, especially if a group of vociferous citizens writes angry letters to the paper. On the other hand, the media have the potential to educate the public about mental illness and its effects, and responsible journalism and televised science programmes can combat ignorance and the prejudice it breeds.

The entertainment media are particularly influential in shaping the public's view of people with mental illness. Nearly three-quarters of mentally ill characters in prime-time US TV dramas are portrayed as violent; over a fifth are killers (Signorelli, 1989). In such Hollywood movies as *Friday the 13th* and *The Silence of the Lambs*, people with mental illness are portrayed as fearsomely dangerous. Mentally ill people are often depicted as bizarre in appearance, vacant, grimacing, giggling and snarling. When the Academy Award-winning film *One Flew over the Cuckoo's Nest* was made at Oregon State Hospital in 1975, the producers had the opportunity to use hospital patients as walk-on actors. They rejected the idea, however, as real patients did not look strange enough to match the public image of mentally ill people (Wahl, 1995). Some more recent films, such as *Shine* and *A Beautiful Mind*, have shown a more realistic and optimistic view of mental illness; and, as we shall see later, advocacy groups have taken on the task of tackling the news and entertainment media about their inaccurate and derogatory portrayal of people with mental illness.

Speaking out

I think 'schizophrenia' is a word that still scares people – professional and non-professional. They think of mass murderers. It still has a bad name. It's like cancer or diabetes used to be. You know, 'cancer' used to be a bad word. I would love to be able to tell my employers, 'Hey, I'm schizophrenic and look at what a good job I'm doing and I'm schizophrenic; isn't that a great thing?' I would like to be able to say, 'Let's celebrate this!'

1.5 Self-stigmatising attitudes

Faced with stigma and prejudice from both the public and mental health professionals, it is no surprise that people with psychiatric illnesses begin to view themselves as inferior to others. They may accept the image that others hold of them as being dangerous and unpredictable. The impact on their self-image is then disastrous, leading to social withdrawal and lack of motivation to achieve their goals. This may be accompanied by depression. The professional attitude to patients with psychotic illnesses is that the more insight they can develop into the nature of their pathological experiences, the better. But for the patients, insight can be very painful, leading to a realisation of how disabled they have become and how much they have lost. Research now suggests that patients who resist the diagnosis of mental illness and who are, therefore, deemed to lack insight have higher self-esteem than those who accept the diagnosis.

Self-stigmatisation

When I got a job I got some criticism, but I didn't tell them I was sick. I didn't want them to know I was mentally ill. I could've been hired as a disabled person because I was mentally ill, but I was embarrassed about the fact that I'd done all these things, and I didn't want anyone to know I was mentally ill. So I never talked about it until just a few years ago. I didn't tell my boss about my history until I got to know her and I wanted her to get to know me as a person rather than for my illness.

1.6 Poverty and social disadvantage

Given the difficulties that people with serious mental illness have in obtaining and keeping jobs, the great majority are on some form of social benefit. Even in the most developed countries, the weekly amounts paid are barely sufficient for the basics of life, and the bureaucratic hurdles to claiming benefits are such that up to half the patients qualified to claim social welfare are not receiving the full amount to which they are entitled (McCrone and Thornicroft, 1997). As a result, patients cannot afford even relatively inexpensive entertainments such as attending sports events or going to the local cinema. Excluded by poverty from participation in such social activities, many patients have no recourse other than to watch endless television, often in a communal setting with other patients, where even the choice of programmes is not under their control.

Lack of money also prevents many patients from buying smart or fashionable clothes, so that their air of shabbiness becomes yet another feature marking them out as different. Some attempt to supplement their income by begging in the street, in competition with mentally healthy but homeless young people, thus becoming identified with the perceived lowest stratum of society.

1.7 Discrimination in housing and employment

Most of the patients who were discharged from long-stay care in psychiatric hospitals were unable to live independently in the community. Consequently, they were rehoused in homes that were staffed during the day and sometimes at night as well. Neighbours who learned that such a home was planned for their street varied in their reactions. The majority were welcoming, or at least accepting, of the new facility. However, a minority often formed determined opposition groups and took political action in order to prevent the home being established. At times, these people were successful and the planned home had to be sited in another locality.

Mentally ill people living in their own homes can be exploited or persecuted, particularly if they live in run-down neighbourhoods, being unable to live in a better environment. Studies have shown that contrary to the public image, people with serious mental illnesses are much more often the victims than the perpetrators of crime.

The difficulties in obtaining work have already been mentioned. These difficulties vary with the economic situation in the area in which the patient lives. When there is a high level of employment, people with a history of mental illness are more likely to find a paid job. However, when unemployment is high, they have very little chance in competition with people without such a history. They are usually more fortunate in agrarian societies with family enterprises, in which they can make a valued contribution, however small, to the family's income.

The working environment offers the opportunity of making friends, gives a structure to the day, increases the person's self-esteem, and provides an income, which enables the person to escape from the poverty trap. All these advantages are denied the person with serious mental illness who cannot find a sympathetic employer.

Discrimination in the workplace

I have to cheat to get a job. I have to make up a past, instead of telling them what's really going on, otherwise I wouldn't get hired. Actually, after I proved that I was a good worker, I once talked to my supervisor about having had a mental problem.

1.8 Human rights

The United Nations issued a Universal Declaration of Human Rights in 1948. Article 22 states: 'Everyone, as a member of society, has the right to social security and is entitled to realization, through national effort and international co-operation and in accordance with the organization and resources of each State, of the economic, social and cultural rights indispensable for his dignity and the free development of his personality.' In the following chapters, we will expand on the themes introduced above, with the addition of remedial action that may be taken to enable the person with serious mental illness to enjoy the human rights guaranteed by the United Nations' Declaration.

Part I

The origins of stigma

The course of psychoses

2.1 The range of course and outcome

Emil Kraepelin (1896) was the first psychiatrist to distinguish between manic-depressive psychosis and what he called dementia praecox, now termed schizo-phrenia. He made this distinction largely on the basis of their different courses, with manic-depressive illness having a relatively benign outcome and dementia praecox, as the name suggests, entailing progressive deterioration. This formula-tion has continued to have its adherents, holding the view that a psychosis that resolves cannot be called schizophrenia. Thus, the fourth edition of the *Diagnostic and Statistical Manual of Mental Disorders* (DSM-IV) of the American Psychiatric Association (1994) stipulates that schizophrenia can be diagnosed only if the symptoms have persisted for at least six months. A condition with exactly the same symptoms as schizophrenia but lasting less than six months is designated schizophreniform psychosis. Earlier diagnostic systems coined a variety of terms for short-lived illnesses with schizophrenic symptoms, including reactive psych-osis, psychogenic psychosis, brief transient psychosis, schizo-affective illness, and the French term 'bouffee delirante'. Guinness (1992) conducted a follow-up study of these transient psychoses in Swaziland and found that some patients relapsed with the same type of transient condition, while between 10% and 20% developed long-standing illnesses that satisfied DSM-IV criteria for schizophrenia. There was nothing in the clinical presentation of the first episode that distinguished between patients with these disparate courses.

Although transient psychotic disorders are less common in developed coun-tries than in developing countries, they do occur. A study of all patients with a psychotic disorder making a first contact with the services over two years was conducted in Nottingham (Singh *et al.*, 2004). The criteria in the International Classification of Diseases, 10th revision (ICD-10) for acute and transient psych-otic disorders (ATPD) with a two-week period of onset were applied to the study sample (World Health Organization, 1992). Thirty-two patients satisfied these criteria. The whole cohort of psychotic patients was followed up for three years and the outcome was compared for the various diagnostic groups. The patients with ATPD fared much better than those with a diagnosis of schizophrenia over the follow-up period. Three-quarters of the patients with ATPD had only a single episode of psychosis or multiple episodes with full remission between, compared with just over one-third of patients with an initial diagnosis of schizophrenia. At first contact, ten of the ATPD patients had symptoms indistinguishable from schizophrenia, and the symptom profile did not predict outcome. This finding confirms that of Guinness (1992) in her study in Swaziland and raises the question of whether these disorders represent a distinct diagnostic category or whether the concept of schizophrenia needs to be extended to include illnesses of very acute onset and rapid resolution.

The international epidemiological study mounted by the World Health Organization, Determinants of Outcome of Severe Mental Disorders (DOSMeD), of patients making first contact with the services for a psychotic illness, substantiated these findings (Jablensky *et al.*, 1992). A two-year follow-up of the samples of patients from a variety of developed and developing countries found that a substantial proportion of individuals with typical symptoms of schizophrenia recovered completely from the first episode of illness and remained well throughout the follow-up period. The importance of these findings cannot be over-emphasised. They demonstrate that schizophrenia is by no means an illness that entails an inevitable deterioration. As we shall see later, the public's stereotype of schizophrenia includes the notion that no one recovers from this illness. Insistence by professionals that only chronic illnesses should be designated as schizophrenia reinforces the public's misconception of the condition.

Even patients with long-standing schizophrenia are not doomed to a dismal outcome. Manfred Bleuler (1978), whose father Eugen introduced the term 'schizophrenia', conducted the first follow-up study of patients with the illness that continued for several decades. Bleuler found that individuals whose illness was unremitting from the beginning showed a tendency to improve as time went on. This surprising result was confirmed by several studies in Europe (Huber *et al.*, 1975; Ciompi, 1980) and a study in the USA (Harding *et al.*, 1987). Some of these patients were considered to have a poor prognosis in the early years of their illness but were found to be working in paid employment decades later.

2.2 Outcome in developed and developing countries

Another key finding from the WHO international study of the onset and course of psychotic disorders was that the outcome over a two-year follow-up was very much better for patients with a first episode of schizophrenia in developing countries than in developed countries. The best outcome was defined as complete recovery from the presenting episode and no further attacks of schizophrenia during the follow-up period. The proportion of patients falling into this category was 24–54% in India, Nigeria and Colombia (mean 37%) compared with 4–32% in developed countries (mean 16%). This is despite the fact that psychiatric resources in India and Nigeria are scarce compared with those in the West. For example, India has four psychiatrists and even fewer psychiatric nurses per one million population (World Health Organization, 2001). Patients with a rapid onset were more common in the samples from developing countries than in the other centres, but even when patients with this type of presentation was excluded the remaining patients fared better than those in developed countries. This makes it unlikely that the explanation lies in the type of illness being compared. It is much more probable that social and cultural differences between the centres account for the varied outcomes. If so, then there are opportunities to alter the patients' environment and, hence, improve their prospect for recovery. This would be an important step in changing the public's conception that people do not recover from schizophrenia.

A long-term international follow-up study has confirmed the findings of earlier long-term studies (Harrison *et al.*, 2001). The sample included 766 of the patients in the DOSMeD study, who were followed up for 25 years. Close to one-half of the patients were rated as globally recovered after this time, and 43% had not been psychotic in the final two years. In terms of social adjustment, 57% of those with a diagnosis of schizophrenia were working in paid employment or were engaged in housework. At an interim 15-year follow-up, 16% of those with schizophrenia showed evidence of late improvement, namely continuous symptoms initially followed by recovery. The overall rates of improvement were found to vary by location, confirming the two-year results, with the best outcomes in Nottingham and rural Chandigarh in northern India.

It would clearly be of practical importance to identify the reasons for the different course of schizophrenia between countries. Several follow-up studies in individual developing countries preceded the WHO DOSMeD study; some of these studies found a better outcome for patients in developing countries than in developed countries. In one study conducted in Sri Lanka, Waxler (1979) suggested that a possible reason was the relative ease with which patients could find useful and productive employment in family enterprises, which abound in rural pre-industrial societies. Waxler's view is supported by a finding made by an earlier WHO transnational follow-up study of schizophrenia (World Health Organization, 1979). These researchers observed that in developed countries it is the best-educated upper-class citizens who have the best outcome in schizo-phrenia, but in the developing world it is the poorly educated farmers who do best. Well-educated upper-caste Brahmins in India, for example, who faced high rates of unemployment at that time, suffered a worse course of illness.

The DOSMeD study was designed to answer the basic question of whether the course of the disease differed between countries and not to look ahead to possible explanations. However, in one of the two Indian centres, the examination of one potential social factor was incorporated – the emotional response of relatives to the development of schizophrenia in a family member. The background to this needs to be introduced.

2.3 Relatives' expressed emotion

A measure of the family's emotional response to schizophrenia was originally developed in the 1960s as part of social research into deinstitutionalisation in the UK. The measurement instrument is known as expressed emotion (EE) and is assessed from an audiotaped interview with the relative(s) (Brown and Rutter, 1966; Vaughn and Leff, 1976). In subsequent decades, EE proved to be a very successful predictor of the outcome of schizophrenia over periods of nine months to two years (Butzlaff and Hooley, 1999). The EE index, which is used to assess relatives' attitudes, is derived from ratings of critical comments, hostility and emotional overinvolvement. It should more properly be termed 'negative ex-pressed emotion', since the expression of warmth by the relative is predictive of a good outcome and does not contribute to the index.

Although the predictive power of EE is remarkably consistent across a wide variety of languages and cultures, the proportion of relatives who fall into the high EE category varies dramatically from culture to culture. It was this observa-tion that prompted the inclusion of the assessment of EE into the DOSMeD study, but only in the Indian centre, as the logistics of this type of research are demanding. Local Hindi-speaking researchers were trained to conduct the inter-views and rate the audiotapes. The patients and relatives were drawn from two different locations, urban and rural. The city of Chandigarh, the capital of the Punjab, is a modern urban environment designed by French architect Le Corbusier. It contains a sophisticated postgraduate medical institute that has attracted professionals from other parts of India; 70% of the population was literate at the time of the study. By contrast, the surrounding villages are popu-lated by traditional peasant farmers, mostly living in mud-brick homes. Here, extended families were the norm, and the literacy rate was 30%.

In terms of EE, 30% of city-dwellers were rated as high, less than half the proportion found by Tarrier *et al.* (1988) in the city of Salford in the UK.

Table 2.1. Proportion of high expressed emotion (EE) relatives across cultures

Country	City	Group	%
Italy	Milan	Italian	70
UK	Salford	British	69
Poland	Cracow	Polish	69
USA	Los Angeles	Anglo-American	67
Spain	Madrid	Spanish	58
Denmark	Aarhus	Danish	54
Australia	Sydney	Anglophone	54
Japan	Okayama	Japanese	46
USA	Los Angeles	Mexican-American	41
Spain	Galicia	Spanish (rural)	34
India	Chandigarh	Hindi (urban)	30
		Hindi (rural)	8

The proportion among the villagers was even lower, at 8% (Wig *et al.*, 1987). Taking the urban and rural relatives together, the proportion rated as high EE was half that of a comparable first episode sample from London, whereas the proportion of patients with the best outcome was double that of the London sample (Leff *et al.*, 1987). The difference in EE levels of the relatives accounted largely for the better outcome of the Chandigarh patients. In order to understand the exceptionally low levels of EE among the Chandigarh relatives, the data need to be viewed in the context of EE studies of other cultural groups, as shown in Table 2.1.

2.4 Variations in EE across populations

It is evident from Table 2.1 that there is a gradient of EE proportions extending from the highest level in urban industrialised populations, through intermediate levels in Mexican-Americans, Western agrarian people and the inhabitants of the city of Chandigarh, India, to the extremely low level found in the rural villagers of Chandigarh province. Low EE represents a tolerant and accepting attitude towards the symptoms and disabilities of schizophrenia, and it appears that this is linked closely to an agrarian economy and the ethos of traditional societies and family structures. We can speculate about the influences that operate in these cultures that may lead to such tolerance.

Family incomprehension

My parents and my sisters were all very 'You're just not using self-control, you're just not trying hard enough, you're doing this for attention.' In fact, my parents are . . . well, rather wealthy, and one time my mother said that if I stopped seeing the psychiatrist, it would be easier for them to afford to bring the maid back from the Philippines. I ignored them and kept seeing my psychiatrist, and they bought their maid back anyway. I have one sister who finally realised that I had an illness. My parents are finally coming around to it.

Beliefs about the causes of illness differ widely between Western and non-Western cultures. In the former, patients are increasingly held responsible for their illnesses; for example, there has been reluctance to offer surgical intervention to heavy smokers with heart disease, since they were considered to have brought the disease on themselves. By contrast, non-Western beliefs about causation entail agents outside the patient's control, such as angered spirits, witchcraft worked against the patient and the operation of fate or karma. Mental illness is ascribed to possession by evil spirits in many traditional cultures, as it was in Europe during the Middle Ages (Leff, 1988). Hence, the patient is not held responsible for her or his illness and criticism by relatives is, consequently, rare.

Another factor that might explain a high degree of tolerance is the pervasive presence of family cooperative enterprises in agrarian economies. The diversity of work roles and the lack of emphasis on productivity and punctuality allow even quite disabled patients to make a contribution to the family income. The inclusion of patients with severe mental illness in the workforce was invoked by Waxler (1979) to explain the good outcome of the patients she studied in Sri Lanka. This is in great contrast to the intensely competitive situation in the West, where late arrival at work and low productivity can lead rapidly to dismissal. A consideration of the sociocultural factors influencing relatives' tolerance of a family member with severe psychiatric illness informs attempts to ease the entry of patients into social and occupational roles in wider society. These will be explored in depth later in this book.

2.5 The nature of negative symptoms

So far, we have discussed variations in outcome in terms of positive symptoms, which delineate new episodes of psychosis when they recur. Negative symptoms differ from positive symptoms in their nature, course and response to treatment. Whereas positive symptoms are marked by the presence of abnormal behaviour and experiences, negative symptoms consist of the absence of normal behaviour.

Conversing with hallucinatory voices and expressing paranoid delusions are typical positive symptoms; not getting up in the morning, not sharing household chores, not washing oneself and not showing interest in anything are characteristic negative symptoms. Unlike positive symptoms, negative symptoms respond poorly, if at all, to antipsychotic medication. Such symptoms generally outlast episodes of positive symptoms by many months and can persist for years.

Negative symptoms give rise to severe social and occupational disabilities and contribute to the public's stereotype of the 'mad' person. Apathy and lack of energy result in neglect of personal hygiene and clothing and lead to a dirty and dishevelled appearance. There is often a restriction or complete absence of facial and gestural expression of emotion, referred to as blunting of affect. People rely so much on smiling to reinforce social intercourse that when it is not forthcoming, there is a disincentive to continue a conversation. Goffman (1963, p. 66) makes the same observation about the effects of blindness: 'the blind person's failure to direct his face to the eyes of his co-participants is an event that repeatedly disrupts the feed-back mechanics of spoken interaction.'

The effects of negative symptoms pervade the social presentation of patients and cause other people to reject them. The effects also influence the attitudes of professionals who try to engage patients in rehabilitation programmes; even though such professionals should be aware that negative symptoms are integral to the illness, they may be critical of them (Moore *et al.*, 1992; Willetts and Leff, 1997).

2.6 The origins of negative symptoms

There continues to be a debate as to the contribution of the social environment to the development of negative symptoms. At the historical turning point of institutional care, a book was published, misleadingly entitled *Institutional Neurosis* (Barton, 1976), which attributed a large part of negative symptoms to the deprived social environment of psychiatric hospitals. It is unquestionable that the 'back wards' of asylums were devoid of stimulation for the patients. If the patients were locked in, their lives were impoverished. However, patients who were free to wander within the walls of the asylum developed their own counterculture, from which staff were excluded and of which they were ignorant. A study of patients' social lives in a psychiatric institution in north London revealed that they had networks of friends and acquaintances outside of the wards, of which the staff were unaware (Dunn *et al.*, 1990). Virtually no social activity between patients or with staff was observed on the wards or in the industrial therapy department. However, a well-developed social community with differentiated roles was observed in the patients' canteen, which staff never entered.

2.7 Does medication worsen negative symptoms?

It is not a simple matter to determine the relative contributions of different influences on negative symptoms, but it is claimed that medication plays a part. The introduction of specific antipsychotic medication in the 1950s offered hope to patients of a return to a more normal life outside of the institutions. However, although the new drugs controlled positive symptoms in a majority of patients, they produced distressing side effects, mainly as a result of blocking of dopamine receptors in the basal ganglia of the brain. This led to a clinical picture closely resembling Parkinson's disease: shaking of the limbs, reduced movement of the face and body, a bent posture and a shuffling gait. Additionally, some patients were afflicted by excessive salivation, with constant dribbling from their mouths. Apart from the distress and discomfort suffered by the patients, these effects on movement and mobility mark out the patients as different and add to the stigma they experience. It has become clear that for decades patients were given much too high doses of these medications. A considerably lower dose than was usually prescribed has been found to completely block the dopamine receptors in the brain, for example 20 mg haloperidol. Additional medication, then, has no beneficial effect on the psychiatric symptoms but increases the frequency of side effects. These unnecessarily high doses also produced sedation, so that many patients had slowed mental processes and some complained of clouding of the mind.

The mental and physical sluggishness resulting from the side effects of medication could easily be mistaken for negative symptoms of the disease. However, unlike true negative symptoms, these side effects resolve when the dose of medication is reduced or when older antipsychotic drugs are replaced with the new generation of so-called novel antipsychotics. As part of an intensive rehabilitation programme in an old psychiatric hospital, Leff and Szmidla (2002) substituted a single novel antipsychotic drug (olanzapine) for the existing regimes. The patients were selected as being among the most difficult in the hospital; many had a history of violence, and some were on an astonishing quantity and variety of medications. One of these medication regimes is shown in Table 2.2.

After their medication regimes were changed, many of these patients became increasingly active and were able to benefit from the rehabilitation programme. As a result, within two years of the start of the programme, 36% were discharged to community placements. Manufacturers of the novel antipsychotic drugs claim that the drugs have a direct effect on improving negative symptoms. This has met with some scepticism from professionals, but a meta-analysis using all available data from the relevant trials, including unpublished material, concluded that there is a basis for these claims (Davis *et al.* 2003).

Table 2.2. Medication regime for one patient in the study by Leff and Szmidla (2002)

Zuclopenthixol[a] 600 mg intramuscular injection weekly
Carbamazepine[b] 200 mg orally four times daily
Chlorpromazine[a] 300 mg orally daily
Chlorpromazine 200 mg orally three times daily
Chlorpromazine 50 mg orally twice daily when required
Haloperidol[a] 20 mg orally at 8 a.m.
Haloperidol[a] 20 mg orally at 6 p.m. when required
Procyclidine[c] 5 mg orally three times daily

[a]Antipsychotic; [b]mood stabiliser; [c]anti-parkinsonian.

2.8 The contribution of institutional practices to negative symptoms

If the deprivation entailed in institutional care is a major determinant of negative symptoms, then one might expect an alleviation of these symptoms once patients are discharged to a more stimulating environment outside the asylum walls. The Team for the Assessment of Psychiatric Services (TAPS) conducted a five-year follow-up study of nearly 700 long-stay patients discharged from two London psychiatric hospitals to homes in the community. A follow-up of the earliest group of 114 patients showed a significant reduction in negative symptoms between the one-year and five-year follow-ups (Leff et al., 1994). However, the five-year follow-up of the entire sample failed to detect any change (Leff and Trieman, 2000). The patients with the least disability were discharged first (Jones, 1993), suggesting that any influence of the institutional environment in increasing negative symptoms is reversible in this group of people. In patients with more severe disability, the institutional effect may be negligible relative to the impact of the illness; alternatively, the institutional effect may not be ameliorated by life in the community. The data do not allow a resolution of these alternative explanations.

The locus of psychiatric care has shifted dramatically over the past 50 years in developed countries. In England and Wales, there were 130 psychiatric hospitals operating in 1975; there are now fewer than 20 still in use. This means that few psychiatric patients are now exposed to the impoverished environments of the past. Sadly, however, negative symptoms have not disappeared with the demise of the institutions. It has become evident that these symptoms are largely a product of psychosis and require specialised treatment in order for the patient to improve. This entails a combination of the most up-to-date pharmacological management and sophisticated psychosocial interventions, as is discussed in detail in Part II.

It must be emphasised that the revolution in psychiatric care that has occurred in Western developed countries has hardly touched the rest of the world. There still exist institutions, even in relatively affluent countries, in which patients live in sickening conditions, wearing nightclothes day and night, tied to beds or chairs, subject to physical assault by staff, and with little hope of returning to their homes. These appalling places continue to dominate psychiatric care and feed the public's image of hopelessness, incurability and alienation.

2.9 Conclusions

There is a wide variation in outcome for people who develop schizophrenia. Although around 15% follow a chronic course from the beginning of the illness, as many as half recover completely from the initial episode and remain well for many years. About twice as many who show this beneficial outcome are found in developing countries as in developed countries, despite the relative lack of professional care in the former. Several explanations have been proposed for this remarkable finding, which is not dependent on the pattern of symptoms at first contact with the services. So far, the explanation that is supported by scientific data is the greater tolerance of family carers in developing countries.

Long-term follow-up studies of people with schizophrenia have revealed that even those who are quite disabled at the start of their illness show improvement in functioning over several decades. However, long periods of hospitalisation impair this tendency to recover, as do excessive amounts of antipsychotic medication. The process of deinstitutionalisation, which has occurred in developed countries over the past half century, has shown that a significant proportion of patients can recover from negative symptoms. This indicates that a socially deprived environment can intensify the apathy and inertia that affect many people with schizophrenia. Other patients fail to find relief from negative symptoms after discharge from long stays in institutions, emphasising the need to avoid such practices. The avoidance of the irrational prescription of medication also has a role to play in facilitating the natural tendency of people with schizophrenia to recovery.

The nature of stigma

3.1 What constitutes stigma?

Most writers on stigma begin by pointing out its linguistic origin in ancient Greece, when the term referred to a brand or scar burned or cut into the body to signify that the bearer was a slave, criminal or otherwise set apart (Clausen, 1981). There is an interesting parallel with the biblical Cain, who, having killed his brother Abel, is marked by God. However, this sign, visible to all who meet Cain, conveys a double message: on the one hand it pronounces him the first murderer, but on the other it declares that Cain, doomed to be a wanderer on the face of the earth, is under God's protection and cannot be harmed by any person. There is a link to the supernatural origin of stigmata and their positive connotation in the use of the term during earlier times to refer to marks resembling the wounds on the crucified body of Christ, which were reported to have appeared on the living bodies of saints and other holy people.

The contemporary usage of the term is entirely negative, as indicated by the subtitle of Goffman's (1963) groundbreaking work on stigma, *Notes on the Management of Spoiled Identity*. Goffman's main argument is that stigmatising attitudes and behaviours by others constitute a threat to the targeted individual's identity. He analyses the different aspects of identity that come under attack, and describes the common responses mobilised to defend one's identity in this situation. It is worth quoting from his perceptive account in some detail.

Goffman distinguishes between three types of identity, each having a different relationship to stigma. Social identity concerns the way in which the individual presents him- or herself to the world at large, comprising people who do not know him or her. Personal identity is the recognition of the individual by the circle of people who know him or her. Ego identity concerns what the individual feels him- or herself to be and, hence, is a personal, self-reflexive experience.

Stigmatisation by others occurs mainly in the realm of social identity and is based on stereotypes held by strangers who are not acquainted with the individual. From this formulation, it follows that people who know the individual are less likely to see him or her in terms of stereotypes and hence to stigmatise the individual. We shall consider the evidence for this proposition below.

Personal identity may be preserved from the effects of stigma by the individual controlling the amount of information imparted to his or her social circle, for example the 'closet' homosexual. A person with a severe psychiatric illness may be able to conceal that he or she has in hospital, but the person's behaviour and appearance may be a giveaway. 'Even where an individual has quite abnormal feelings and beliefs, he is likely to have quite normal concerns and employ quite normal strategies in attempting to conceal these abnormalities from others, as the situation of ex-mental patients suggests' (Goffman, 1963, p.156). This can also be true of current psychiatric patients, who learn quickly of the adverse consequences of admitting to professionals the extent of their abnormal experiences. I (JL) used to sit in my office in an old psychiatric hospital, overlooking the verandah of a villa in which lived 12 long-term patients, for whose care I was responsible. One elderly man, who had been an inpatient for many decades, used to sit on the verandah talking loudly to thin air and laughing uproariously. Whenever I saw him in my office to review his mental state, he would deny vigorously that he heard voices.

Patients can learn from each other how to cope with stigma and to maintain their personal identity. People who share the same stigmatised characteristic can provide the individual 'with instruction in the tricks of the trade and with a circle of lament to which he can withdraw for moral support and for the comfort of feeling at home, at ease, accepted as a person who really is like any other normal person' (Goffman, 1963, p.32). However, some individuals – and this is certainly true of psychiatric patients – do their best to distance themselves from others of their kind.

The stigmatised individual tends to stratify others with the same stigmatising characteristics according to how apparent and obtrusive is their problem. He can then take up the same attitude to the more evidently stigmatised as 'normals' take to him . . . Presumably the more allied the individual is with normals, the more he will see himself in non-stigmatic terms.

Goffman, 1996, pp. 130–31

Goffman points out that the person who develops a stigmatised characteristic later in life (as with most psychiatric illnesses) will be faced with the possibility of accepting a new identity. One advantage of succeeding in this is access to support from others with the same stigma. But there is the need to cope with the grief at losing 'normal' status. The damage to self-esteem that this loss entails has been the focus of increasing research and will be discussed below.

3.2 Public attitudes towards psychiatric illness

There have been many surveys of the public to determine their attitudes towards people with psychiatric illness. This is not a simple matter of asking questions, because the way in which questions are asked can influence the answers. People are often aware of the 'correct' answers to give and may respond as they believe the questioner would like them to. This is known as a socially desirable response, which can lead to a wide gap between people's reports of their attitudes and what they secretly believe. People also respond differently to an open-ended question such as 'How would you recognise someone with a mental illness?' compared with a suggested characteristic such as 'Do you think people with mental illness are likely to be violent?'

In addition, it is instructive to discover how well informed people are about psychiatric illness, since prejudiced attitudes often stem from ignorance. Attitudes do not necessarily correspond with actual behaviour, and so it is also necessary to ask people how they would behave towards a mentally ill individual. Once again, there can be a disparity between what people say they will do and how they behave in reality. Therefore, a comprehensive enquiry in this area will include questions about knowledge, attitudes and behavioural intentions. There should also be some check on how people actually behave towards mentally ill patients in real-life encounters. This is a demanding programme and few studies have been so inclusive.

One method of minimising socially desirable responses is to present to members of the public case histories of mentally ill patients without giving a diagnosis. Vignettes of this kind were first introduced by Star (1955) and have become a common tool with which to explore attitudes. There is a large literature on attitude surveys using vignettes or questionnaires, or both. We will not attempt to review all published studies, but we will focus on representative research and studies that have added new understanding.

3.3 Findings from surveys

Reda (1996) conducted an attitude survey in two streets in north London and asked an open-ended question about the characteristics of people who were mentally ill. The 68 people in one street who responded and the 60 people in the other street identified the same characteristics and in almost exactly the same order of frequency. Poor communication was mentioned by 41% and 36%, respectively, closely followed by strange behaviour (32% and 39%). Poor social skills were next in frequency, followed by aggression, which was mentioned by 22% and 17%, respectively. These proportions are surprisingly low in view of the media representation of mental illness, to which we have referred above. However, surveys that ask directly about mental illness and violence find a much higher proportion of the public endorsing this supposed link.

Crisp *et al.* (2000) used the Office of National Statistics (ONS) to conduct a face-to-face survey of 2679 adults in the UK from random addresses. Questions were asked about seven mental disorders, including schizophrenia. The proportions ascribing various characteristics to schizophrenia were as follows: unpredictable, 77%; danger to others, 71%; hard to talk to, 58%; feel different, 58%; never recover, 51%; not improved if treated, 15%; need to pull self together, 8%; and only themselves to blame, 8%. The contrast with Reda's results is striking: in Reda's survey, unpredictability was the least frequent response in one street, while in the other it was more often identified than aggression, which was the least commonly mentioned response. It is improbable that such differences are due entirely to the local nature of Reda's sample compared with the national survey. The different techniques of assessing attitudes constitute the most likely explanation.

Reda (1996) also found that the level of knowledge about mental illness was low, with 35% of respondents being unable to distinguish between mental illness and learning difficulty. A similar lack of understanding was found by Wolff and colleagues (1996a) in a survey of 215 residents of two areas in south London. As many as 48% of respondents could not make the distinction between mental illness and learning difficulty. A national survey in the UK was carried out at about the same time as Wolff *et al.*'s study and included a representative quota sample of 1804 adults aged over 15 years (Leff, 1998). Each respondent was presented with a list of illnesses and asked to identify which of them were mental illnesses. Thirty-two per cent stated incorrectly that learning difficulty was a mental illness. The mental illness recognised by most (85%) respondents was schizophrenia, although 44% thought it meant a 'split personality'. As in the local London surveys, only a small proportion (14%) identified schizophrenia with violent or aggressive behaviour.

A telephone survey by Stuart and Arboleda-Florez (2000) in Alberta, Canada, revealed a high level of understanding. Only 10% of respondents thought that people with schizophrenia tend to be mentally retarded or of lower intelligence. A relatively low proportion (18%) ascribed dangerousness to people with schizophrenia. Respondents over the age of 60 years had a less enlightened view of schizophrenia and its treatment. Those people who were the most knowledgeable were the least likely to distance themselves from people with schizophrenia. Despite the well-informed nature of the Canadian public, 47% of respondents equated schizophrenia with split personality.

The German public also understand schizophrenia in terms of split personality (Angermeyer and Matschinger, 1997); this association is commonly found in studies of what Jorm *et al.* (1997) have termed 'mental health literacy'. Schizophrenia is derived from the Greek words *schizo* (meaning split) and *phrenos* (meaning mind), but few members of the public, outside of Greece, would be aware of its linguistic roots. We need to seek another explanation for this widespread misconception.

The whole range of psychiatric disorders attracts some degree of stigma, but schizophrenia is viewed by the public as the second most dangerous condition, substance abuse being first. Both the public and the media interpret schizophrenia as denoting split personality, with associated images of Dr Jekyll and Mr Hyde. Robert Louis Stevenson's novel was actually a sophisticated argument for the recognition that every person is subject to aggressive impulses and that we are constantly suppressing these as a result of being socialised. But the idea of splitting them off ('hydeing' them) and, thereby, becoming a perfectly calm and rational being is illusory. Each of us is an uncomfortable mixture of the good doctor and the passionate beast. And yet the need to deny our violent passions and to label them as 'madness' is both profound and pervasive. Sontag (1988), writing about cancer, proposed that 'diseases acquire meanings (by coming to stand for the deepest fears)'. The process of ridding ourselves of the feared urges to be violent and impulsive is achieved only by attributing these unwanted characteristics to others. The despised other then becomes someone we wish to extrude from civilised society. This was, of course, the fate of hundreds of thousands of people with psychiatric illnesses who were admitted to asylums and often spent the rest of their lives isolated from the outside world.

This formulation underlies a number of the questionnaires employed in community surveys. For example, a factor analysis of the Community Attitudes to the Mentally Ill (CAMI) scale devised by Taylor and Dear (1981), which has been used widely, yields three factors, two of which are 'fear and exclusion' and 'social control' (Wolff *et al.*, 1996b). Respondents scoring high on the first factor express considerable fear of mentally ill people and wish to extrude them from society. Those with high scores on the second factor endorse measures to exert greater control over people with mental illness. The third factor is in contrast to the other two as it represents 'goodwill', a set of attitudes that is gratifyingly common among the public, as we shall recount later.

> ### Stigma at the university
>
> This teacher always seems to be complaining about me, that I'm intruding on her, that I'm invading her space. I got feedback from my other teacher that this was happening. Last year, this teacher taught the continuing education class in the evening and she recommended that I enrol in a regular class in the spring. When I did that, she called the campus police, and the police called me at my house and said I was to have no connection with her. Not to call, not to speak to her, not to go to her classes, not to write, have nothing at all to do. I didn't know why. She must have heard from somebody, somewhere, that I have a schizophrenic diagnosis. For people in society, schizophrenics are very scary people. So she became afraid of me that I was going to cause her some harm or something. That does not help to have somebody in a position of authority, a teacher at a university, talking behind your back to other teachers, saying things like, 'You have to watch out for this person.'

3.4 Stereotype versus reality

If stereotyping involves assigning to people with mental illness those aspects of ourselves that we disown, then are we simply projecting shadows on to a blank screen or is there some substance to the stereotype? Data that allow us to examine this question were collected by the TAPS in the course of evaluating the transition from psychiatric hospitals to community care. Patients staying more than one year in two London psychiatric hospitals due for closure were assessed comprehensively before their discharge or death. Excluding patients with dementia, 670 patients were examined, which included an interview with staff to ascertain their severe behaviour problems (Sturt and Wykes, 1986). The commonest problem of this kind was poor hygiene and appearance (74%), followed by underactivity (52%), lack of initiative (26%), incoherence of speech (22%), inability to make appropriate social contact (22%), and poor concentration (22%) (O'Driscoll *et al.*, 1993).

The severe communication problems affecting one in five of the patients assessed by TAPS provide some basis for the stereotype held by the public. In Reda's (1996) survey and the ONS national survey (Crisp *et al.*, 2000), respectively 40% and 58% of respondents considered that people with schizophrenia are difficult to communicate with. However, in relating the stereotype to the actual problems presented by this sample of users, it is essential to recognise the context of the TAPS study. The two psychiatric hospitals concerned had been reducing the size of their patient population since the mid 1950s. By the time the TAPS survey was conducted in the late 1980s, the hospital populations had shrunk to one-third of their peak size. The better-functioning patients had been discharged (Jones, 1993), so that the residual population studied by TAPS comprised the most disabled patients. Even in this group, only a small minority displayed the problems of communication that form part of the public stereotype.

3.5 Mental illness and violence

We have seen that the proportion of the public endorsing dangerousness when asked directly was 71%. Does this reflect the reality of violent acts committed by mentally ill people? This is not a simple matter to elucidate, because the most violent group in the general population consists of young men, and the group in which schizophrenia first manifests itself is young people, with men having an earlier onset than women. Therefore, in comparing the rate of violent incidents in people with schizophrenia and the general population, it is essential to control for age and sex.

Angermeyer (2000) reviewed the nine epidemiological studies of violence and mental illness published since 1990. He found a moderate but significant relationship between schizophrenia and violence. However, a much higher risk of violence was associated with substance abuse and with antisocial personality disorder. Arboleda-Flórez (1998) noted from a review of the literature that substance abuse is a significant risk factor for violence and criminality among the community, patients and offender populations alike. He also pointed out that violence by patients is frequently directed at family members and friends and usually occurs at home. Thus, the fear of members of the public of being attacked in the street by a psychiatrically ill person has only a slender basis in reality. Furthermore, violent acts are committed by only a small minority of former patients.

This observation is supported by findings from the TAPS study. The five-year follow-up of 670 long-stay patients discharged to the community found that 13 patients committed assaults on members of the public (Trieman *et al.*, 1999). These individuals slipped through the selection net set up by hospital staff to identify patients who could be aggressive and who were then referred to secure facilities. To put the figure into perspective, assaults were committed by 2% of the patients over a five-year period.

Taylor and Gunn (1999) examined homicides by mentally ill people in the UK over the period during which the locus of care shifted from psychiatric hospitals to community-based services. They found no obvious increase in such homicides over time. Furthermore, they noted that homicides by mentally ill people form a very small proportion of all homicides. To summarise, only a tiny proportion of mentally ill people commit violent crimes, only a very small percentage of homicides are perpetrated by mentally ill people, and family members and friends are much more at risk than strangers from assaults. Taking this summary into account, it is clear that the perception of the majority of the public that mentally ill people are generally dangerous is greatly exaggerated.

It is evident that the negative image held by the public of mentally ill people is based on the characteristics of a very small and unrepresentative group. One of the users interviewed by Wahl (1999) pleaded: 'Don't take the most severe form of mental illness and say that's the way it is for everybody.' Generalisation from the worst affected patients to all mentally ill individuals is the basis of the process of stereotyping. We will now examine the factors that shape the attitudes of the public and may lead to stereotyping.

3.6 Factors influencing attitudes

Sociodemographic factors

The respondent's age, social class and level of education have regularly been found to influence attitudes towards mentally ill people. Older people usually express more need to exert control over psychiatric patients (Rabkin, 1974; Taylor and Dear, 1981; Brockington *et al.*, 1993; Wolff *et al.*, 1996b). As this finding has been consistent for more than 20 years, it is unlikely to be a cohort effect but rather suggests that people's attitudes harden with age. Some light is thrown on this by Angermeyer and Matschinger (1997), who found that respondents with more traditional values, such as achievement, duty, acceptance and materialism, expressed the desire for greater distance from mentally ill people.

More tolerance towards mentally ill people is expressed by people of higher occupational level (Taylor and Dear, 1981; Brockington *et al.*, 1993) and by better-educated people (Cumming and Cumming, 1957; Maclean, 1969; Brockington *et al.*, 1993). Wolff and colleagues (1996b) examined the associations between sociodemographic variables and the three factors derived from the CAMI by factor analysis, namely 'fear and exclusion', 'social control' and 'goodwill'. People with high scores on the 'fear and exclusion' factor tended to be older and of lower occupational level, confirming previous findings. This was also true of people with high scores on the 'social control' factor, who in addition were of lower social class. A novel finding from this study was that people with children under the age of 18 years in the household had higher scores both on 'fear and exclusion' and on 'social control'. The authors felt that this was related to the stereotype of mentally ill people as representing a serious threat to children, for which there is no factual basis. A greater preference for social control was also shown by ethnic

Asians, Africans and Caribbeans. An analysis of the relationship of attitudes to knowledge of mental illness (Wolff *et al.*, 1996a) showed that respondents who wished to see more social control had less knowledge of mental illness. This was particularly true of older respondents, those of lower social class, and members of ethnic minority groups.

People with high scores on 'goodwill' were younger and better-educated, while low scores were linked with membership of an ethnic minority group. Eighty per cent of respondents knew of somebody who had a mental illness, and this was associated with less endorsement of the need for social control. This observation raises the question of the degree to which contact with mentally ill people influences attitudes.

Contact with mentally ill people

The earlier research produced contradictory findings, but results from more recent work have been consistent. Rabkin *et al.* (1984) studied the attitudes of people in New York living close to mental health facilities and used a comparison group that had no such facilities locally. The majority (77%) of experimental residents were unaware of the facility in their neighbourhood, while 13% of the control respondents incorrectly identified such a facility as being located near them. All respondents were asked whether they thought that 'mental patients treated in the community are a danger to people in the area'. Only 27 (15%) people agreed with this statement; of these, 25 said they were unaware of living close to a facility, although in fact 14 of them did so. The authors concluded that experience is not a determinant of the belief about the dangerousness of mentally ill people. This does not seem a valid conclusion, since few of the neighbours living near a facility were aware of it and presumably had little or no contact with the patients.

Reda (1995) conducted a similar study in London, surveying the neighbours of a residence for discharged long-stay patients and comparing their attitudes with those of residents in a parallel street. She found that few of the experimental neighbours recognised the nature of the residence, and those that did so assumed that it was a home for senior citizens. This was not so surprising, since the average age of the patients was around 60 years.

It is clear that reliance on casual contacts with mentally ill people is an uncertain strategy for exploring effects on attitudes. Link and Cullen (1986) conducted two random surveys of community residents, one in Macomb, Illinois, and the other in Cincinnati, Ohio. They found significant negative correlations between the amount of reported contact with mentally ill people and perceived dangerousness. The association was not explained by sociodemographic variables known to be associated with attitudes towards mentally ill people. One possible interpretation is that people who have little fear of mentally ill people seek contact with them. To investigate this possibility, Link and Cullen divided contacts into those chosen by the respondent and those dictated by uncontrollable circumstances. Even in the latter type, more contact reduced fear of mentally ill people. Therefore, it seems that contact produces more favourable attitudes. This conclusion was supported by Angermeyer and Matschinger (1996), who conducted two population surveys, one in western Germany in 1990 and the other in unified Germany in 1993. They found that willingness to interact socially with a person with schizophrenia increased with greater intensity of exposure to mental illness. In a subsequent series of surveys, Angermeyer and Matschinger (1997) confirmed this for both schizophrenia and depression.

In a recent extension of this research, Link and Phelan (2004) undertook telephone interviews with 1507 adults in the 20 largest cities in the USA, achieving a response rate of 63%. Respondents were asked about the perceived danger of mentally ill people, the degree of personal contact (people known personally), the degree of impersonal contact (mentally ill people seen in public places), and experiences of being threatened or physically harmed by someone who had been hospitalised for mental illness. Greater contact was associated with lower perceived danger and also with greater exposure to threat or harm. Not surprisingly, those who had been threatened or harmed were more likely to perceive mentally ill people as dangerous. Nevertheless, these associations did not result in an overall positive association between contact and perceived danger. Exposure to threat or harm accounted for only 1% of the attributable fraction of perceived danger. A fairly large proportion (around one-quarter) of fearful perceptions was attributable to personal characteristics of the respondents that were unrelated to their exposure to threat.

Link and Phelan (2004) conclude that their findings imply that removing people from public view or controlling their symptoms with medication will not be enough to eliminate rejection and discrimination. The way to tackle fear and social control must, then, include addressing the personal issues that generate these attitudes.

Do attitudes differ with diagnosis?

We have noted above that the public are not well-informed about the distinctions between diagnostic categories in psychiatry. Nevertheless, some conditions attract greater stigma than others. A few researchers have compared the attitudes of the public to different psychiatric conditions. Angermeyer and Matschinger (1997) used Link and colleagues' (1999) Social Distance Scale in 11 population surveys in Germany. They presented to subjects five case histories depicting schizophrenia, major depression, alcohol dependence, panic disorder with agoraphobia, and narcissistic personality disorder. Each respondent was presented with only one vignette. Alcohol dependence produced the greatest social distance, followed by schizophrenia and then personality disorder. Greatest social acceptance by far was for major depression and panic disorder. This was confirmed for employers by Manning and White (1995), who sent out questionnaires to 200 personnel directors of public limited companies. They found that there was much more tolerance for applicants with depression than for applicants with schizophrenia.

As part of a campaign against the stigma of mental illness run by the Royal College of Psychiatrists in the UK, Crisp *et al.* (2000) used the ONS to conduct a national attitude survey. Questions were asked about seven mental disorders: severe depression, panic attacks, schizophrenia, dementia, eating disorder, alcohol addiction and drug addiction. Schizophrenia, alcoholism and drug addiction were the most negatively viewed disorders. Drug addiction was seen as more dangerous to others than schizophrenia. This reflects the reality of the differential risk as assessed by Angermeyer (2000), based on his review of the literature, and shows that in this instance the public perception is accurate.

We learn from this small group of studies that there is a spectrum of stigma for psychiatric conditions, with substance abuse being most heavily stigmatised, followed by schizophrenia and personality disorder. The neuroses, including depression and anxiety states, are the least stigmatised, probably because they are so common in the general population and are not associated with violent behaviour.

Variation in attitudes by country

The World Psychiatric Association mounted a global programme, which has been in existence since 1996, to reduce the stigma and discrimination of schizophrenia. The scientific director of this programme is Norman Sartorius, and to date 20 countries are participating. One of the initial steps in developing a programme locally is to conduct a survey of public attitudes to direct the focus of the programme. Ideally, each country should use the same survey instrument, but in practice this was difficult to achieve. However, there is sufficient similarity in the questions asked to allow comparisons to be made between nine of the countries involved in the earlier stages of the global programme.

Table 3.1 summarises the responses to 12 questions, showing the countries' ranking in terms of the most positive and the most negative responses to each question. There is a marked consistency in the appearance of specific countries in the two columns. Canada, Germany and Poland dominate the most positive attitudes column, while the most negative attitudes column features almost exclusively Greece, Japan, Macedonia and Turkey. The exceptions are Austria, with the worst attitudes to working with a psychiatric patient (although Greece

Table 3.1. Ranking of centres across questions

	Most positive	Most negative
Reaction to a group home in neighbourhood	Germany	Macedonia
Schizophrenia = split personality	Poland	Greece
Schizophrenia = mentally retarded	Canada	Japan
Treatability	Poland	Turkey
Can be treated in the community	Canada	Macedonia
Seen talking to self or shouting in street	Canada	Greece
Need prescription drugs	Greece	Japan
Dangerous to others	Germany, Canada	Greece
Public nuisance due to begging, poor hygiene	Germany	Greece
Can work in regular jobs	Japan	Greece
Would work alongside a patient	Canada	Austria, Greece, Turkey

and Turkey tie for second place), and Japan, with the most positive attitudes to patients working in regular jobs. This anomaly for Japan may result from the strong work ethic that is characteristic of the Japanese culture and Japan's high level of employment.

It is noteworthy that the list of questions includes knowledge about schizophrenia, attitudes to psychiatric community care, optimism/pessimism about outcome and preferred social distance. The sample sizes in these surveys ranged from 100 (Macedonia) to over 7000 (Germany), and it is striking that there is such consistency in ranking, indicating that there is a coherence between knowledge, beliefs and attitudes.

In considering what we can learn about the determinants of stigma from these findings, it is necessary to state that we can only speculate at this stage. Our hypotheses should form the basis of more detailed enquiries involving the countries concerned. If we ask what Canada, Germany and Poland have in common, they are industrialised countries with comprehensive systems of state health care, which have progressed towards a reduction in size of their psychiatric institutions and development of community psychiatric services. By contrast, psychiatry in Greece, Turkey, Macedonia and Japan remains centred on the psychiatric hospital. In fact, Japan is unique among developed nations in increasing the number of psychiatric hospital beds in recent years in contrast to the general trend of reduction. Furthermore, almost all Japanese psychiatric hospitals are privately owned and run and consequently are not under government control. The rights of mentally ill people in Japan are poorly safeguarded, and until recently a law allowed family members to lock a patient within the home if they considered he or she to be suffering from a psychiatric disorder.

The psychiatric hospitals in Greece, Macedonia and Turkey generally provide a poor standard of care. The hospital on the island of Leros in Greece became an international scandal when the inhuman conditions there were exposed. One of us (JL) visited what was reputedly the best of the four psychiatric hospitals in Macedonia. It was undoubtedly one of the worst in the author's experience, with one ward shared by psychiatric patients and patients suffering from chronic tuberculosis.

The link between hospital-centred care of a poor standard and repressive attitudes of the public towards psychiatric patients can be interpreted in two ways. It is possible that the high visibility of closed institutions from which few patients return reinforces the public's stereotype of madness as dangerous and incurable. Norman and Malla (1983) found that the belief that mental illness has a poor prognosis was correlated with greater social rejection. Alternatively, the persistence of such institutions is a manifestation of general societal attitudes towards psychiatric illness. As with most dichotomies of this type, the truth probably lies between the extremes, favouring an interactional model. This means that closing down the old asylums and replacing them with community services that have low visibility is likely to ameliorate negative public attitudes.

Stigma in the mental health centre

I met with this one therapist a few times and I just felt like she was talking to me like maybe I was retarded, or the way you would talk to a foreign person who doesn't speak English too well. She spoke a bit slow, so I found that a bit aggravating.

3.7 Self-stigmatisation

Attitudes of professionals and relatives

Patients have to face rejecting attitudes not only from the public, which can be dealt with by social withdrawal, but also from family members and the professionals from whom they seek help, which are less easy to avoid. Jorm *et al.* (1999) surveyed members of the Australian public, general practitioners (GPs), psychiatrists and clinical psychologists. The psychiatrists were the most pessimistic about the long-term outcome of schizophrenia. By contrast, a recent survey by the Royal College of Psychiatrists in the UK showed that psychiatrists were more optimistic about recovery from schizophrenia than the general public (Kingdon *et al.*, 2004). Nevertheless, only one-quarter of the psychiatrists responding to the questionnaire thought that a full recovery from schizophrenia is possible. A likely explanation for this is that patients with schizophrenia who recover well from their first episode drop out of contact with the psychiatric services. Thus, the patients with schizophrenia that psychiatrists see regularly are biased towards chronicity. Lefley (1987) surveyed mental health practitioners who had personally experienced long-term major mental illness in their own families. Most of the relatives were not comfortable discussing mental illness in the family with colleagues. Only 26% indicated they would feel free to talk about the situation, and another 26% expressed strong reluctance; the remainder said they would disclose to only a few people who they thought would understand.

Given this degree of reluctance to disclose among mental health professionals who are also informal carers, it is not surprising to find even greater reticence among non-professional family members. Phelan *et al.* (1998) interviewed 195 parents or spouses of patients with psychosis. Half of the relatives reported some attempt to conceal the patient's hospitalisation. Almost 40% either told no one or limited communication to close friends, neighbours and family. Concealment was greatest among parents not living with the patient, family members with higher educational attainment, and relatives of female patients.

Karidi and colleagues (2006) in Athens developed the Self-Stigma Question-naire for users. They gave this questionnaire to a random group of 150 outpa-tients with a diagnosis of schizophrenia or schizo-affective psychosis. The users reported that 58% of their family members kept the illness secret from relatives, 47% from close friends and 33% from neighbours. This kind of reaction is also seen in non-Western cultures. Shibre *et al.* (2001) conducted a study in Ethiopia, in which relatives of patients with schizophrenia or affective disorder were asked questions on stigma, beliefs about illness and coping mechanisms. Of the re-spondents, 80% lived in rural locations and 77% were illiterate. At least one answer on stigma was positive in 75% of cases. Over one-third (37%) felt the need to hide the illness, and 17% made an effort to keep it secret.

Thara and Srinivasan (2006) interviewed family carers of 159 outpatients with schizophrenia in Chennai, India. The users' mean duration of illness was 12 years. Slightly more than half the primary caregivers were men, a reversal of the proportion in the West; over half of the caregivers were parents. The main worry for 55% of the carers was the marriage prospects of other family members. This reveals how in Indian culture, the stigma of the patient's illness casts its shadow over the whole family. Consequently, 38% of carers worried that people would find out about the patient, 37% worried that neighbours would treat them differently or avoid them (32%), and 36% expressed a need for concealment. However, it was almost impossible to hide the patient's illness, and those who discussed it with neighbours received more help and understanding than those who concealed the illness.

Family incomprehension

My mother thought I was never mentally ill. She never accepted that. She said, 'Oh, you're just having problems.' I had to accept there's certain things I can't talk about with my mother because she won't understand. You don't talk about feelings in front of her. She never thought I was sick, no matter how many hospitals. No matter that I pulled a knife on her when I was sick and went to jail.

Impact on self-esteem

Concealment by family members perpetuates stigma by not sharing information with other relatives and friends. It also deprives them and the patient of support from their social networks. The effect on the patient is that he or she feels that what has happened to them is unmentionable, giving a damaging blow to self-esteem. Professionals value the patient who accepts that he or she is ill, as this is considered to facilitate compliance with treatment. But accepting that one has a serious psychiatric illness casts gloom over one's future and can also lower self-esteem. Kennard and Clemmy (1976) have shown that psychiatric patients undergoing treatment in which the emphasis is on confronting the reality of the illness status show changes to their self-concept. Patients who were given a diagnosis of schizophrenia or paranoid psychosis underwent a change from a positive to a negative self-image during the course of their admission.

Labelling theory and its modification

The deleterious effects of a psychiatric diagnosis were formulated as labelling theory in the 1960s (Scheff, 1966), which became one of the central tenets of the anti-psychiatry movement. In essence, labelling theory postulates that unusual beliefs and behaviours that are innocuous in themselves are labelled as pathological by psychiatrists, condemning the individual to an unmerited career as a patient. In other words, the label of a psychiatric diagnosis creates a pathological state in the person. This view has become increasingly untenable with the discoveries of a biological basis to the psychoses, but Link and colleagues (1989) have modified labelling theory in an attempt to rescue it from the dustbin of outdated ideas. It is worth quoting their reformulation of the theory verbatim:

Once labelled, an individual is subjected to uniform responses from others. Behaviour crystallises in conformity to these expectations and is stabilised by a series of rewards and punishments that constrain the labelled individual to the role of a 'mentally ill person'. When the individual internalises this role, incorporating it as a central identity, the process is complete and chronic mental illness is the consequence.

These authors reject the idea that labels create mental illness directly, but they suggest that labelling and the consequent stigma can lead to a poor outcome for the person. They reiterate Goffman's (1963) analysis of the possible responses to stigmatisation, namely secrecy, withdrawal and attempting to educate others (see Section 3.1). They also point out that 'each of these responses limits patients' life chances'. The result is that 'many patients will lack self-esteem, social network ties, and employment as a consequence of their own and others' reactions to labelling'.

Discrimination in the workplace

There is a stigma about going to see a psychiatrist. You're supposed to be strong and be able to work through your problems . . . not taking all this medication and not being able to pull your weight. There is a stigma, and when I go to work I don't tell them I'm a mental health patient. If I have problems, I explain it then, but I don't bring it up with my co-worker and my boss. I just don't want them to know my past, that I've had problems, because then they'll think it'll interfere with your work and they won't hire you. You can call it discrimination, but they're not going to take a chance with somebody they know has a mental illness over someone who doesn't have a mental illness.

Effects on lifestyle and choices

Link *et al.* (1989) find evidence for their predictions from a survey of psychiatric patients and healthy community residents. Patients with more concern about stigma were more reliant on household members for practical support. The greater their fears of stigma and devaluation, the less practical support was available from non-household members. These findings of reduced social networks were consistent across two diagnostic groups, schizophrenia and major depression.

The difficulty experienced by people with a history of psychiatric illness in finding a job has been discussed above. At first contact with the psychiatric services, at least half the people given a diagnosis of schizophrenia are unemployed (Mallett *et al.*, 2002). This is not simply a result of their disability. A national survey of employment in the UK found that only 13% of people with a history of psychiatric disorder were working compared with over one-third of disabled people generally (Office of National Statistics, 1998), demonstrating that discrimination against mentally ill people by employers must be occurring. This is confirmed in the USA by the users surveyed by Wahl (1999), 33% of whom reported that they had been turned down for a job for which they were qualified after their mental health consumer status was revealed.

The effect of stigmatisation on the patient is expressed vividly by Gallo (1994) from her personal experience. She defines self-stigmatisation as a process 'whereby mentally ill individuals torture themselves to an extent that exceeds what they suffer from the very worst that society-at-large can dish out to them'. She was labelled as 'chronically mentally ill' after a single acute psychotic episode in 1985, from which she recovered:

I tortured myself with the persistent and repetitive thought that people I encountered, even total strangers, did not like me and wished that mentally ill people like me did not exist . . . I now realize that (my neighbours) perceived me as being stand-offish and rejecting of them because of my own self-imposed reclusive behaviors . . . I was acutely aware of how terribly narrow and limited choices can be when one passively accepts self-stigmatization.

Discrimination in the workplace

I just wasn't performing like I had in the past, so I was fired. Maybe they should've waited until I recovered and gotten a temporary employee in there and then waited until I recovered and let me get my job back. They could've been a little more understanding. I was too embarrassed to tell them what I was going through, so they thought I was . . . they knew I wasn't acting right and I didn't go to them with . . . telling them about it. So it could've been better both ways.

Self-esteem and depression

In her account, Gallo (1994) confirms the restriction of choice that self-stigmatisation imposes. There is clearly a depressive tinge to her perception of how she is viewed by others, reflecting the strong association between low self-esteem and depression. Link *et al.* (1997) studied a group of 84 men with dual diagnosis of severe mental illness and drug/alcohol abuse who were enrolled in model programmes for treatment of these conditions. Link *et al.* measured three components of the stigma process: culturally induced beliefs about devaluation and discrimination, experiences of rejection, and ways of coping with stigmatisation. At baseline, perceived devaluation/discrimination and rejection experiences were associated significantly with depression, unlike the stigma-coping methods of secrecy and withdrawal, which were unrelated to depression. A year later, the pattern of associations was unchanged. Men who remained in the treatment programme for a year improved substantially in psychiatric symptoms. However, there was no decline in the perception of stigma, in stigma-coping methods or in the recall of rejection experiences. This suggests that depression is a response to stigma rather than depressive symptoms increasing the perception of stigma. Depressive symptoms constitute a significant problem for users, 14% of whom in Wahl's (1999) survey complained of persistent anxiety and depression.

Insight and self-esteem

The evidence indicates that there are negative consequences, in terms of lowered self-esteem and depression, to accepting the professional opinion that one is mentally ill. Is the reverse true? Warner *et al.* (1989) studied 42 patients with psychosis and found that those who denied they had a mental illness reported higher levels of self-esteem, regardless of the extent to which they stigmatised mental illness. Patients who acknowledged that they had a mental illness had lower levels of self-esteem if they perceived mental illnesses to be highly stigmatised. However, those who accepted the label had relatively better functioning. A study by Morgan (2003) provided confirmation of the link between self-esteem and insight. His subjects consisted of an epidemiological sample of patients making first contact with psychiatric services for a psychotic illness and a group of controls from the general population. Patients with a diagnosis of depressive psychosis or schizophrenia had significantly lower self-esteem than the controls. Lower self-esteem was associated significantly with greater insight and with increased compliance with treatment. This study shows that self-esteem is already below that of healthy people at the inception of schizophrenia and of depressive psychosis. In the latter illness, low self-esteem may well be an integral part of the depressive syndrome; however, in schizophrenia, it is possible that it is an early response to an awareness of the stigma attracted by a severe mental illness. The findings of Warner and colleagues (1989) make it clear that it is the patient's perception of stigma that leads to lowered self-esteem.

Stigma in the workplace

I've never said anything about my illness to anyone at the store where I work. I get the sense that they may not be very understanding. I think that I would probably have problems if I said anything. One time, one of the people there was angry about her son's girlfriend and she said, 'I think she's a schizo.' She didn't mean 'I think she's got schizophrenia'; she was just using that as an expression. So, it's just a place that I would never, ever, say anything.

Concealment and its causes

In Wahl's (1999) survey of users, nearly 80% had overheard people making hurtful or offensive comments about mental illness, 77% encountered hurtful or offensive media portrayals on at least some occasions, and 60% had experienced being shunned or avoided. Interviews with 100 of the users surveyed revealed that the commonest source of stigma was the community, followed by relatives and then professional carers. The perceived stigma from professionals was their pessimistic attitude to possible achievements. These adverse experiences led 57% of users to report lowered self-esteem and loss of confidence. Such experiences also made the users less likely to disclose information about themselves, more likely to avoid social contact, and less likely to apply for a job or educational opportunities.

Revealing one's mental illness

I don't tell people right away that I'm mentally ill. I consider that's right up there with starting out on your religion or telling about a gallstone operation. You get to know somebody and after a while you tell them. If the subject comes up, I'll tell them, but I have to get to know somebody before I tell them. The people I tell just say, 'Oh, that's interesting', and some will ask me a little about it, and some just won't be interested in it. But I never tell employers. It's not something to tell an employer.

Confirmation and extension of these findings has come from the groundbreaking study by Karidi and colleagues (2006) of self-stigmatisation by people with schizophrenia in Greece. Nearly half these subjects had been ill for more than ten years and 78% had been hospitalised. In answer to a question on concealment by their family, 58% reported that their illness was kept secret from relatives, 47% from close friends and 33% from neighbours. The greater openness with neighbours was presumably because of the difficulty in hiding the illness from them. Thirty-three per cent of the users said that they did not feel comfortable talking about their illness to anybody, just over half thought that if others knew about the illness the response would be fear, and two-thirds thought that they would be avoided. From their experience, 59% reported avoidance by friends, 53% insults from people, and 40% the expression of fear by people.

In response to being asked about the most painful experience in their life in relation to their illness, 64% gave no answer. The rest of these Greek users (consumers) cited the negative attitudes of others, giving as examples the use of violence, beating and swearing. These punitive actions may surprise us, but they are matched by the findings of a postal survey conducted in the UK by the voluntary organisation Mind (1996). Of the 778 respondents, 47% had been abused or harassed in public and 14% had been physically attacked. Harassment was severe enough to force 26% of respondents to move house. Among the Greek users, the prevailing feelings identified as a result of being stigmatised were hopelessness and feeling disregarded and downgraded by others. Those who had never been hospitalised reported better acceptance by relatives and friends than those who had been admitted to hospital.

A recent survey in a general hospital in south-west England compared users on psychiatric wards with those on medical wards (Bromley and Cunningham, 2004). The users were asked how many of their family members and friends they had told of their admission and how many they had informed about their diagnosis. Significantly fewer of the psychiatric users than the medical users told family members of their admission, and they were even less likely to tell extended family members or friends. The diagnosis was disclosed to family by 63% of psychiatric users and 95% of medical users. The proportions who told their friends their diagnosis were 55% and 90%, respectively. Psychiatric users gave a variety of reasons for concealment, which stemmed mainly from their experience or fear of stigma by others. Examples cited by the authors include 'People will always be watching me afterwards' and 'People are afraid: they judge you differently when they know'.

The response to a schizophrenic illness of 'sealing over' is categorised as an avoidant coping strategy (Thompson, McGorry et al., 2003). A study of the factors associated with sealing over found no link with a negative view of the self, confirming Morgan's (2003) results, but a strong relationship with the belief that others view them in a negative way (Tait et al., 2004). From the research findings and personal accounts, the predominant strategies employed by users against stigma are social avoidance and concealment, or limited disclosure. However, in Wahl's (1999) survey, a minority responded by speaking up and attempting to educate people who made disparaging or incorrect statements about mental illness.

Speaking out

I have to worry when I speak out because there's too much stigma. I just had a letter about mental illness printed in the local newspaper. I had to worry about my two employers seeing it, because they don't know that I have schizophrenia. If they knew, one of them I think would be accepting, but the other one I don't think would be.

3.8 Users' needs for acceptance and personal growth

A study explored the neglected area of users' views of what they want from family, friends and professionals, and their existential needs (Wagner and King, 2005). Interviews were conducted with users in a Brazilian city who were receiving psychiatric care for schizophrenia, and with their informal and formal carers. Focus groups were held regarding the topic of users' needs, and qualitative analysis of transcripts was conducted.

The majority of users had experienced discrimination, to which they responded by a wish to withdraw and conceal themselves. They craved respect and expressed the need to be understood. They recognised that when they felt useless, incapable or insane, they were internalising the prejudice of others. They often perceived others as indifferent or averse to them. One user summed up this experience as 'nobody wanted to have a relationship with a schizophrenic'. Some commented on the need to control their sense of shame and anger and to respond appropriately when they were discriminated against.

Many felt that they had lost the achievements they valued and saw the illness as a malign obstacle to their personal development. They suffered intensely from the feeling that their physical and emotional integrity was constantly in danger of fragmenting. Some complained that their relatives and doctors interpreted everything they experienced as madness rather than a threat to their sense of identity and humanity.

Although some users did not accept the diagnosis of schizophrenia, others recognised that acceptance of the illness was an important existential need, regardless of whether it had any 'meaning'. Many felt that adequate information about the nature of their illness helped them to question their symptoms, challenge them and progress. The findings of this study emphasise the importance of listening to the users' experiences of the disorder and the responses of others to them, and the value of giving them full information about the illness.

3.9 Conclusions

The public's stigmatising attitudes to people with psychiatric conditions are based on stereotyping, which flourishes when there is inadequate knowledge, misconceptions, and little contact with mentally ill people to correct them. Secrecy by family members and pessimistic attitudes of professionals perpetuate stigma. The effect on users is to lower self-esteem and induce depression. Users can defend themselves against these negative effects by denying that they are ill, but that strategy has its own deleterious consequences through non-compliance with treatment. Social withdrawal and concealment are also common strategies employed by users, which incur penalties in the form of loss of support from their social networks. Users feel keenly the rejecting attitudes of others and tend to internalise the negative image held by the public and disseminated by the media. The courageous user who opts for disclosure and/or attempts to educate prejudiced people can do very little single-handed. As we shall see, however, it is possible to change public attitudes and to reduce social distancing by education, but this needs to be done by collaboration between users and enlightened professionals.

The old-style psychiatric hospital projects the image of incarceration and incurability, which reinforces the public's stereotyped image. The policy of replacing hospitals with community psychiatric services will contribute to a reduction in stigma. However, realising the policy produces new problems, which will be considered in Chapter 8.

Poverty and social disadvantage

4.1 The two populations of users

In discussing the effects of poverty and social disadvantage on people with severe psychiatric disorders, we need to distinguish between two populations. One population comprises those users who have spent a considerable period of time in psychiatric hospitals and have been resettled in the community. In developed countries that are phasing out psychiatric hospitals, this population is diminishing in size and will eventually become inconspicuous relative to the other population. This other population comprises those users who may have been admitted to psychiatric wards in general hospitals but who have never spent years of their life in institutions. Both populations may be subject to poverty and social disadvantage, but in the long-stay group these factors are compounded by the deleterious effects of institutional life on employment prospects, social networks and the accretion of stigma. These effects are interactive, since the stigma attached to a long admission to a psychiatric hospital weighs heavily against finding a job, lack of employment constrains finances and diminishes the possibility of expanding social networks, and years spent in an institution destroy existing social networks.

There is a new group of long-stay users emerging who spend over a year in the psychiatric wards of general hospitals. However, this experience is not comparable with decades incarcerated in an isolated psychiatric hospital that family and friends are reluctant to visit. The bulk of the literature on social networks relates to the traditional long-stay users, so we will consider them separately from current users.

4.2 Social networks of long-stay users

The environment within the old psychiatric hospitals was one of social deprivation, made worse by the users' progressive loss of contact with relatives through death or reluctance to continue visiting. The TAPS survey of the social networks of long-stay users in two London psychiatric hospitals found that three-quarters of the 505 responders to the Social Network Schedule had no contact with any relative (Leff *et al.*, 1990). Although the staff were unaware of much of the users' social activity off the wards, the users did have established social networks, albeit small in extent. On average, each user could name two people they considered to be friends, but one-fifth could not identify anyone they would call a friend. Over two-thirds included no members of staff in their network, despite the long tenure of many of the staff in the hospital. Setting relatives aside, over 90% of users had no contacts in the community.

This depiction of the users' social networks will strike many readers as bleak compared with their own circles of friends and acquaintances. However, the reality is probably even starker, since 24% of users in the study were unable or unwilling to complete the Social Network Schedule while in hospital. In addition, we have evidence from other assessments that those who refused to complete the Social Network Schedule were more socially disabled than those who cooperated. Half the users had been in hospital continuously for over 20 years, which may have been responsible for a considerable depletion of their networks. Whatever the explanation, the quantity and quality of the networks did not augur well for social reintegration of these users into the community.

4.3 Social networks of people with schizophrenia over time

It is important to discover whether the networks of people with severe psychiatric illness attenuate over time, regardless of stay in hospital. Lipton and colleagues (1981) tackled this issue by delineating the social networks of 15 people with schizophrenia on first admission and 15 who had a history of schizophrenia for more than two years and had been admitted to hospital at least once in the past year. It emerged that the size of the networks of long-term users was less than half that of first-time users, with a mean of 6.3 compared with 15.5. The long-term users had fewer contacts who were non-relatives than did the first-time users. The intensity of relationships was diminished greatly among the long-term users: one-third did not have a very good friend, a very close contact or a very important person in their lives, whereas first-time users had significantly more of all of these. Only two individuals in each group reported having no close friends in their teenage years. Hence, it appears that most of the reduction in size of the social networks of people with schizophrenia occurs after their first admission.

Lipton and colleagues (1981) consider that the nature of the changes in the social networks combined with the users' self-reports indicate that the causes are not solely the social deficits stemming from schizophrenia. Rather, there is likely to be a contribution from the avoidance of the user by non-relatives. As we have seen above, this is typical of stigmatising attitudes towards people with schizophrenia. Lipton *et al.* suggest that educating the families and friends of users early on in the illness might help to maintain the integrity of their networks.

4.4 Changes to the networks of users discharged to the community

The TAPS study of long-stay users resettled in the community included follow-ups at one year and five years after discharge from the two psychiatric hospitals. After one year of living in the community, there was no change in the size of the users' networks, but there was an improvement in quality (Anderson *et al.*, 1993). A significant increase occurred in the number of people considered to be friends: on average, each user gained one extra friend. This may not sound much of an advantage, but it has to be appraised in the context of very small networks containing an average of two friends. A small number of the new friends were neighbours of the users, raising the question of how far the users were able to integrate socially within their new neighbourhoods.

The majority (78%) of these long-stay users were discharged to staffed group homes; 7% went to unstaffed homes and 15% were able to live independently. It is conceivable that the users in staffed homes were surrounded by a cordon sanitaire of professional carers who insulated them from contact with ordinary members of the public. To investigate this possibility, we defined a category of social contact, which we termed an acquaintance, who was neither a user nor a provider of psychiatric care. There was an increase in the proportion of users who knew at least one acquaintance, from 19% in hospital to 29% in the community. Most acquaintances were met at social clubs or were neighbours, or relatives and friends of carers, so some users made social contact with ordinary citizens but they still represented a minority of those discharged from long-stay care. Part of the problem undoubtedly lies with stigmatising attitudes of the public.

At the five-year follow-up, there was still no change in the size of users' networks, but there was a further increase in quality (Leff and Trieman, 2000). The number of friends remained the same, but there was a significant increase in confidants. A confidant was defined as a person to whom the user could tell their troubles and, hence, represents a more intimate relationship than simple friendship. It is natural that it took longer for the users to acquire new confidants than to form additional friendships.

4.5 The social mix in community homes

Although a minority of users were able to break out of the circle of mental health users and providers, most were trapped within it. This does not necessarily sentence them to an impoverished social life, since users can provide each other with friendship and company. However, this depends on the severity of social disability affecting the individuals selected to live together in the same residence. A comparison of the social networks in two residences studied in the TAPS project showed that in one residence, intense and reciprocated relationships developed over time. By contrast, in the other residence, the individual users remained relatively isolated from each other, with no increase in the intensity of their mutual relationships (Dayson, 1992). The largest contribution to this failure to gel was that the users selected to live in the second residence had almost all been social isolates in the hospital and lacked the capacity to establish reciprocal relationships. One user in a different programme described this problem clearly: '[the residence] would have been alright if it had acted as a community, but everybody was very isolated and although we might go for a drink with somebody from time to time we didn't function as a house – it was individuals living close together but isolated' (Barham and Hayward, 1996). The solution suggested by Dayson is that users chosen to live together should represent a balance of socially able people and those who lack the ability to make social contact with others.

4.6 The social life of users in a community-based service

Negative symptoms and social withdrawal

We can now consider users who have never spent long periods of time in psychiatric hospitals. In countries that have instituted community care, users are not exposed to the socially deprived environment of the old remote hospitals that deterred friends and relatives from visiting. Nevertheless, users can still experience a restricted social life due to a number of factors. We have discussed above the nature of negative symptoms and have argued that they are an integral part of schizophrenia, although undoubtedly they are intensified by institutional environments; such symptoms include restriction of emotional expression through the voice, the face and the use of gesture. The consequent lack of responsiveness in social interchanges discourages others from communicating with the affected individual. Social withdrawal is usually included among negative symptoms, but it differs from symptoms in being an active response by users to situations they find difficult to tolerate. Social withdrawal appears to be a defensive strategy employed when users feel highly aroused by a social encounter (Tarrier *et al.*, 1979).

It is illuminating to consider here an unusual piece of qualitative research undertaken in a psychiatric hospital in the UK that specialised in rehabilitation of users referred from other hospitals. Morgan (1979) ran a small group for users with schizophrenia who were the most severely disabled people in the hospital, having failed to benefit from an intensive rehabilitation programme. Twenty-five users attended the group during an average of four years. They had been ill for a mean of 21 years, most of that time being spent in a psychiatric hospital. Morgan analysed the content of discussions from notes kept over the course of the group. He found that the topics of greatest interest for users were food, money, smoking and sleep. Most users knew the amount of their weekly earnings; half made their income last the week, but others were insolvent within two or more days. Most money was spent on consumables, especially cigarettes, tea, sweets and beer. Only a few users ever bought new clothes or other possessions.

Morgan recorded that 'one topic that was invariably unpopular with the group was current events. They signified their hostility by yawns, resigned-looking grins, and silence, thereby generating considerable group tension and discomfort'. Most of the users did nothing on their holidays from work. 'They welcomed a holiday from work but had no idea what to do with it . . . They resented my efforts to stimulate them into activity and usually reacted with mute hostility . . . I realised, and sympathised with, their lack of unlimited money, of transport and of family or friends to prompt them into activity.'

Morgan concluded: 'The keynote of their various disabilities was poverty. There was evidence in most cases of social, cultural and material poverty in their original upbringing. Clinically, there was poverty of intellect, affect and volition.' He considered that the disabilities were due to schizophrenia rather than institutionalism and that 'such chronic schizophrenic patients (will become) no less disabled outside hospital after a similar length of illness'.

The psychiatric hospital in which Morgan worked, St Wulstan, was the first in the UK to close. His prediction has been borne out by subsequent experience of the emergence of users with chronic disabling schizophrenia in the absence of psychiatric hospitals. Unfortunately, a small proportion of people never recover from a first attack of schizophrenia and suffer from persistent psychotic symptoms for the rest of their life. The DOSMeD study of the WHO (Jablensky *et al.*, 1992) revealed that 10–15% of people making first contact with the services for a schizophrenic illness experienced no relief from their symptoms throughout a two-year follow-up. This proportion was much the same regardless of the country in which the individuals lived. Given the wide range of cultures represented in this study, it is a reasonable assumption that this type of treatment-resistant schizophrenia is the least responsive to the social environment. This does not mean that we have to be pessimistic about the social and occupational integration of these users, but clearly they will need specialised and protracted professional efforts in order to achieve these aims.

Effect of stigma on the family's social network

We have already described the stigma felt by family carers of people with severe psychiatric illnesses (see Section 3.7). The common response is to withdraw from their own social networks. Carers stop going out to visit relatives and friends and no longer invite people into their homes. This has the dual effect of losing the support available from their network and considerably restricting the user's social circle. It has been shown that families with a psychiatrically ill member have networks of a normal extent at the start of the illness, but that these shrink progressively as the illness persists (Anderson *et al.*, 1984), mirroring the reduction in the users' networks over time (Lipton *et al.*, 1981).

Healthy siblings of the user may respond to the illness by distancing themselves as far as possible from the user, moving out of the home or spending as much time away as they can. In Western industrialised and urbanised societies, the extended family of traditional cultures has been replaced by the nuclear family, but this is now under threat through the high divorce and separation rates. It is not uncommon to find a middle-aged user being cared for by an elderly mother, with no other relatives in touch with the couple. The isolation of the couple is intensified if the parent is overinvolved with the user, maintaining an exclusive relationship with him or her.

4.7 The location of residences for users

The social activity of users living apart from their families is influenced by where they live. The opportunities for any newcomer to a neighbourhood to make friends depend on the character of the area and the strength of the sense of community. Run-down neighbourhoods with high levels of crime, vandalism and drug-dealing are the worst places for mentally ill people to live. Users with severe psychiatric illnesses are particularly vulnerable to harassment and victimisation. The TAPS study found that long-term users were more often victims than perpetrators of crime (Trieman *et al.*, 1999). Furthermore, the ready availability of street drugs puts users at risk for relapse of their illness. Unfortunately, opposition to the opening of residences for users tends to be most forceful in pleasant, suburban, middle-class neighbourhoods, where people cite a feared drop in property values as one of their main objections. In the public attitude survey conducted by Wolff *et al.* (1996b), 15% of respondents agreed with the statement 'Residents have good reason to resist the location of mental health services in their neighbourhood.'

Campaigns of a 'not in my backyard' (NIMBY) nature are often waged by a small but vigorous minority of residents who express prejudiced attitudes, stereotyping mentally ill people as dangerous and unpredictable. Some of these campaigns have successfully prevented residences for users being established in pleasant areas, forcing the planners to locate the residences in less desirable neighbourhoods. However, a nationwide survey in the UK of providers of mental health services revealed that there was no regional variation in the frequency of opposition (Repper *et al.*, 1997). Of the organisations responding to the survey, all three national voluntary organisations, six of the seven housing associations, eight of the nine health service trusts and 65% of the local voluntary organisations had faced opposition in the previous five years. Local opposition ranged from protest letters, through meetings, to violence directed at property, users and staff. This kind of reaction led to 30% of local voluntary organisations abandoning plans altogether.

In planning the siting of residences, a major consideration has been to avoid the creation of ghettos, leading to a concentration of large groups of users in the same area (Lamb, 1983). However, there is an awareness of the logistic advantages of a small group of residences arranged close to a central facility for day care, the so-called 'core and cluster' model. This affords users easy access to structured activities and also enables staff to circulate around the residences, thus reducing the number of staff required.

In the initial phase of planning accommodation in the community for the long-stay users in two north London psychiatric hospitals, the emphasis was on new-build housing. This was soon abandoned on the grounds of expense and replaced by the conversion of existing properties. The latter proved to be a better option for the users, because, as we have seen above, buildings that are indistinguishable from others in the street do not advertise their function as sheltered housing and are often not recognised by neighbours as accommodating mentally ill people.

4.8 Availability of daily activities

In the UK, the most disabled patients are housed in staffed homes, generally providing a good standard of accommodation and meals in addition to security of tenure (Trieman *et al.*, 1998a). However this is not universally the case in Europe and North America. In the USA, the main provision for long-term users unable to live independently is known as 'board and care'. Lamb (1979) sought the opinions of residents and staff in board-and-care homes about these facilities and found that some regarded the operators as treating them solely as a business, squeezing out excessive profits at the expense of the users. In fact, board and care developed into a major industry with an annual turnover of $16 billion, large enough to attract the attention of the Mafia (Brown, 1985). A small number of homes provoked public scandals when it was discovered that the greed for profit led to residents being housed in inhumane conditions and fed inadequately.

Budson (1983) described how in the USA during the 1970s, legal actions ('class actions') were brought against state mental health systems, which resulted in legally binding standards of care in the psychiatric hospitals. This led to 'economically motivated discharges'; however, there were too few appropriate community residences in order to cope with the number of discharged patients. Very many 'drifted into proprietary boarding homes and single occupancy hotels into a kind of isolation that was little better than that of the hospital wards'. The problem was compounded by the lack of structured daily programmes. Budson (1983, p.290) was also critical of board-and-care homes, some of which 'provide little more than room and board in dingy surroundings, with no semblance of a rehabilitation program whatsoever'.

In Britain, deinstitutionalisation also involved some undesirable practices. During the 1970s and 1980s, the opportunity was seen to place discharged long-stay patients in seaside boarding houses. These are usually empty and close down during the winter. The offer of permanent residents all year round was seized on by the owners. However, there is little to do in a British seaside resort during the winter, since almost everything shuts down, and no programmes of activities were laid on for the residents (Barnes and Thornicroft, 1993). Television documentaries presented bleak images of users in raincoats wandering along deserted rainswept promenades, and the exposure of this shoddy practice led to its discontinuation.

4.9 Homelessness

The high visibility of homeless mentally ill people on city streets inevitably reinforces the public stereotype of the 'mad' person, since many of them are dirty, unkempt and strangely dressed, and they are often seen to be shouting, talking or muttering to themselves. We need to enquire into the causes of homelessness among people with psychiatric illnesses, as identification of these could lead to preventive measures.

It is difficult to gain an accurate estimate of the number of homeless people in a city because of the many places in which they find shelter, including derelict houses, abandoned cars and doorways. A homeless user who came under the care of one of us (JL) used to hide in a laundrette until the automatic time lock secured the door at night. This example reveals the streetwise skills that users can acquire in order to survive in the hostile environment of inner city streets. Since the 1970s, surveys of homeless people in residential settings have estimated the prevalence of severe psychiatric illness (excluding alcoholism) at between 25% and 45% (Leff, 1997). Kovess (2002) came to a similar conclusion from her review of the literature, estimating the lifetime prevalence of psychiatric disorders among homeless people as ranging between 28% and 37%. She also concluded that substance abuse and the absence of family support are key factors contributing to homelessness among people with psychotic disorders.

Caton and colleagues (1994) conducted a case–control study of homeless men with schizophrenia; they found that homelessness followed the onset of the psychosis in one-third of the men. This gives some hope of preventing the slide into homelessness in at least this proportion of men with schizophrenia. Studies of the childhood histories of homeless people identify a high prevalence of institutional care (Bassuk, 1984). This is often the result of parental neglect and/or physical and sexual abuse leading to the child being taken into care. The applicability of this observation to homeless mentally ill people was elucidated by Sullivan *et al.* (2000), who compared homeless people with and without psychiatric illness. Both groups were similar in terms of demography and the experience of considerable poverty in childhood. However, the homeless people with a psychiatric illness comprised a higher proportion who had been taken into care as children, who had suffered sexual or physical abuse in childhood, and who had a primary caregiver who was mentally or physically disabled. Herzberg (1987) studied homeless people with a psychiatric illness and found that half the sample had a history of separation from parents of more than three years' duration.

These findings suggest that disruption of parent–child relationships has a destructive effect on the ability to form stable bonds with others in later life, and that when a psychiatric illness supervenes the additional dislocation of ties leads the individual to seek the anonymity of a vagrant life on the streets. It would require a massive campaign to reduce child physical and sexual abuse, but there are encouraging signs that this is beginning in some countries. A law has been instituted in the UK that limits the amount of physical chastisement that a parent can give a child. Furthermore, an increasing awareness of the prevalence of sexual abuse of children and its damaging effects in producing adult mental illness has led to the establishment of telephone lines via which children can report abuse.

For users who are living with their families when the illness begins, conflicts with relatives in the household can result in ejection or voluntary departure of the user from the home. Work with families of users with severe psychiatric illness has proved effective in reducing conflict and promoting problem-solving skills

(Kuipers *et al.*, 2002). Therefore, the instigation of work with families as soon as a diagnosis of a severe psychiatric illness is made in one of the members may avoid some users from embarking on the path that leads to social isolation and homelessness.

4.10 Poverty and quality of life

As we have seen, over half the users with severe psychiatric illness at their first contact with the psychiatric services are unemployed. As the illness progresses, the problem worsens: the unemployment rate for users in the UK with long-term illnesses exceeds 85% (Office of National Statistics, 1998). The situation is somewhat better in Italy, which has a higher level of employment among users (Warner *et al.*, 1998). Many developed countries have established a welfare system that grants benefits to people with long-term illnesses. In the UK, there is a disability allowance; in the USA, there is a disability pension. However, these benefits are not generous compared, for example, with those given in Scandinavian countries, and it is difficult for users to maintain a reasonable quality of life on benefits. Bradshaw *et al.* (1992) studied the economic status of a number of households in the UK. They found that by 1991, the value of social security benefits had declined below the level required to purchase adequate food and clothing.

There have been surprisingly few studies of the financial problems of people with severe mental illness living in the community. Some information on these can be gleaned from research evaluating the quality of life of these people. Rosenfield (1992) studied 157 users of a clubhouse in New Jersey, based on the Fountain House model. She requested users to complete Lehman's (1988) Quality of Life Scale. A large percentage of those who reported that work was the most important part of the programme to them stressed that it was the hope or chance that they would find work that was critical. Services for financial support were related significantly to quality of life. Combined with the findings on vocational rehabilitation, help with securing economic resources is viewed by users as making a major contribution to life satisfaction.

Sullivan *et al.* (1991) also used Lehman's Quality of Life Scale, from which they selected questions to pose to users with schizophrenia who had been discharged from Mississippi State Hospital. Most of the 101 subjects were African-Americans who lived in rural areas or small towns. Their responses were compared with those from samples of seriously mentally ill people studied by Lehman and colleagues and with those from a national sample of non-mentally ill people. The scores of the Mississippi sample were significantly lower than those of the national healthy sample in the areas of finances and social life. Compared with subgroups of the national sample who were of low socioeconomic status or were black, the Mississippi users were more dissatisfied with finances and social life. Comparison with Lehman's samples of seriously mentally ill people from Los Angeles and from Maryland showed again that the Mississippi users were less satisfied with their finances. The Mississippi sample was the only one comprising people residing primarily with family members. Most were relatively poor: in almost one-half of the households, no family member had been employed in the previous year. It is possible, therefore, that the families' lack of resources exacerbated the users' financial position.

Data on the association of severe mental disorders and poverty were obtained from the second British National Psychiatric Morbidity Survey, which was carried out between March and September 2000. A clinical interview was undertaken with those respondents who passed a screening interview for psychosis for the definitive identification of psychotic conditions. It was found that psychotic disorder was 17 times more common in those earning between £100 and £200 a week, and 35 times more common in those earning under £100 a week, compared, with those earning over £500 a week (Jenkins, personal communication, 2005). As well as indicating their income, respondents were asked whether they had incurred different types of debt over the last year. One-third of respondents with a psychotic condition were in debt compared with 12% of the general population (Jenkins, personal communication, 2005). The most commonly reported debts were for council tax, telephone, rent, gas, water, electricity, TV and mail-order payments. One in ten respondents with a psychotic disorder had had their telephone disconnected due to debt, with obvious implications for their ability to make social arrangements. Around a third of people with psychosis borrowed money, the main sources for borrowing being family and friends.

Poverty

I do have enough money to survive, but it pisses me off that I'm almost 40 years old and I'm not saving any money and I live at such a low standard of living in my peak earning years. It really upsets me. I'm thankful that I don't have any children that I'm putting through poverty.

4.11 Conclusions

Long-stay users in the old psychiatric hospitals pose particular problems for integration because of the deleterious effects of custodial care on their social networks, their initiative and activity, and their knowledge of the world outside the institution. Nevertheless, an increase in the quality of their social networks can take place after they have spent some years in the community. However, relatively few of these users have been able to establish relationships with ordinary citizens.

The problem of long-term disabilities will not vanish with the demise of the psychiatric hospitals, as new chronic users are arising from the population. These users will need focused and protracted programmes to help them overcome their social and occupational disabilities.

The social networks of users and their family carers begin to shrink with the onset of the illness, constituting a strong argument for early intervention in order to preserve their natural support networks. Sheltered housing for users not living with relatives needs to be sited in neighbourhoods that have low levels of crime and substance abuse. Opposition to such residences is usually mounted by a small minority of the public, who can be neutralised if the goodwill of the majority is mobilised. Once a residence is established, opposition tends to melt away. Wherever users live, daily structured and unstructured activities should be within easy reach, either by foot or by a single means of public transport.

Homeless mentally ill people are conspicuous on the streets of many cities and reinforce stigmatising attitudes. Homelessness needs to be tackled by preventive measures focused on the control of child physical and sexual abuse and psychological help for children separated from their parents for whatever reason.

The majority of people in developed countries who suffer from severe psychiatric illness are without work. Welfare benefits are insufficient to make up the loss of earnings and are reduced when users start to earn from sheltered work. Many unemployed users are supported by their families, who make financial sacrifices to do so. Very low incomes and debts for basic amenities are common among people with severe psychiatric illness. Lack of money affects a user's ability to make new social relationships, since he or she is prevented from enjoying leisure activities that could bring them into contact with their peers. The absence of a job also reduces the possibility of increasing their social networks. Ways of tackling the issues around employment are the subject of Part II.

Ameliorating users' symptoms

5.1 Optimising medication

We have argued in previous chapters that psychotic symptoms that are untreated or that do not respond adequately to treatment increase stigma, since such symptoms reinforce the public's stereotype of the mentally ill person. Additionally, both positive and negative symptoms interfere with the user's ability to engage in work and social activities. The first line of treatment is pharmacological, but this has its own deleterious effects on users' functioning. The most disabling side effects of conventional antipsychotic drugs are parkinsonism, sedation and sluggish thinking. The parkinsonian effects result from blocking of the dopamine-2 receptors in the basal ganglia of the brain. The new-generation antipsychotic drugs have a different pattern of action. They block the effect of dopamine for much briefer periods of time than the standard antipsychotic drugs (Kapur and Seeman, 2001) and they also have a blocking action on the effect of the neurotransmitter serotonin (Sartorius et al., 2002).

The most effective of the so-called atypical antipsychotics is clozapine, but this has the potentially lethal effect of suppressing white cells in about 1% of the people receiving it. Therefore, it is essential to test the blood regularly in clozapine users to check the number of white cells. Some clozapine users refuse to have their blood tested, meaning that they should not take this drug. Other atypical antipsychotics in common use include risperidone, olanzapine and amisulpride. The blocking effect of risperidone on dopamine-2 receptors increases substantially at higher doses, so it is advisable to keep the dose low.

Brain-imaging studies have shown that in the past, far too high doses of antipsychotics were given routinely, producing unnecessary side effects. For instance, a dose of 20 mg haloperidol completely saturates the dopamine receptors in the brain, and so there is no therapeutic gain in giving any more than this over 24 hours. Positron-emission tomography (PET) scans show that clinical improvement occurs when 65% of dopamine-2 receptors are blocked by medication and parkinsonian side effects occur when 78% of these receptors are occupied (Kapur and Seeman, 2001). Users are likely to get optimal benefit, therefore, when doses are kept well below 100% receptor occupancy. It used to be common practice to increase the dose of a drug to the maximum recommended dose and then, if psychotic symptoms persisted, to add another antipsychotic drug without stopping the first one. As a result, users received excessively large amounts of antipsychotic medication and were heavily sedated. The term 'chemical straitjacket' was applied to this practice. It was seen most often in psychiatric wards catering for long-stay patients with persistent psychotic symptoms, particularly in patients with a history of aggression. The combined effects of the excessive medication and the socially deprived environment made it unlikely that such users would be considered for discharge to the community (Trieman *et al.*, 1998). However, replacing such regimes of multiple conventional antipsychotics with a single atypical antipsychotic improves the ability of users to participate actively in rehabilitation programmes and enables a good proportion of users to leave the psychiatric hospital (Leff and Szmidla, 2002).

Cognitive coping strategies

There is one thing that I developed for myself that I've been doing for at least ten years. When the voices get really bad and are arguing too much, I'll pick a phase and I'll just repeat it over and over so that I don't join in the arguments. One of my favourite phrases is 'Oh! Weather the weather, whatever the weather, whether I like it not.' I'll just repeat this over and over again, and it calms me down and tells me, 'Don't join in with the arguments. I'm just going to carry on no matter what.' I'll pick a word that I really like the sound of, like 'Shostakovich'. I'll just repeat 'Shostakovich' over and over, like a mantra. The voices will be arguing in the background. I can still hear them, but I'll tend not to join in because I'll be paying attention to saying the word I chose. I still do this every night.

    It's sort of an acceptance of the way things are. Accepting that there are voices in my head and I can't do anything about it. Not trying to fight, because I know I can't win. I found this out by myself because I realised I couldn't stop the voices. No medication would stop them. I mean, if I were to take enough medication to stop the voices, it'd make me too gaga to function. But if I said one of my phrases over and over, I calm down. I realised that when I would join in with the arguments, it led nowhere. They never decided anything of importance. They would just argue about maybe what TV channel to watch. So I learned to say, 'Whatever'. Like, 'OK, you go ahead and decide whatever you want to do, decide whatever you decide and I'll go ahead and do what I want to do. Whatever the decision is, I'll do what I want to do anyway.'

Even with the best drug treatment possible, there remains a proportion (about 40%) of users whose psychotic symptoms are not dealt with adequately and remain very troublesome to the users and their family carers (Marder, 1996). These patients include those who fail to recover from the first episode of psychosis (see section 2.9). The recent introduction of cognitive-behavioural therapy (CBT) for psychosis has offered the hope of improving the quality of life of these users.

5.2 Cognitive-behavioural therapy for psychotic symptoms

Since the 1990s, a number of randomised controlled trials of CBT for psychotic symptoms have been published. Tarrier and colleagues (1993; 1998) conducted two trials, the first with users who had drug-resistant psychotic symptoms and the second with users who had chronic schizophrenia. In the first trial, users who were trained to enhance their strategies for coping with psychotic symptoms improved significantly more on a measure of delusions than those who were taught problem-solving. In the second trial, CBT produced a significantly greater reduction in the number and severity of psychotic symptoms than supportive counselling.

Kuipers and colleagues (1997) studied users with psychotic symptoms that were resistant to medication and compared CBT with standard care. At a nine-month follow-up, users assigned to CBT showed a significantly greater improvement across the range of psychiatric symptoms than those in the standard care group. However, the changes in delusions and hallucinations did not reach significance. At an 18-month follow-up, the improvement in the CBT group was maintained at much the same level as that recorded at nine months, and a highly significant improvement in distress caused by delusions and a significant reduction in the frequency of hallucinations emerged (Kuipers *et al.*, 1998).

Sensky and colleagues (2000) also focused on users with schizophrenia and randomised them to either CBT or befriending by a therapist. At a nine-month follow-up, CBT produced a significantly greater improvement in all symptoms measured compared with befriending. Two trials have addressed users with an acute episode of psychosis. Drury and colleagues (1996) compared cognitive therapy with a control intervention involving the same amount of time spent on recreation and informal support. Both groups of users experienced a decline in positive symptoms, but this was significantly greater in the experimental subjects. Negative symptoms declined equally in both groups and were negligible by the twelfth week of the study. At a nine-month follow-up, the users who received cognitive therapy showed significantly fewer positive symptoms than the control group.

A trial in the Netherlands focused on inpatients with schizophrenia who had residual delusions or auditory hallucinations after at least three months' treatment with medication, including an atypical antipsychotic (Valmaggia *et al.*, 2005). The patients were randomised to CBT or supportive counselling. After 16 sessions of treatment, patients who received CBT showed a significant improvement in auditory hallucinations, but not in delusions, compared with those in the control group. However, the difference between the two groups was no longer evident at a six-month follow-up.

This brief review indicates that CBT is efficacious in reducing delusions and hallucinations in both chronic and acute psychoses. It is particularly valuable for users whose psychotic symptoms are controlled inadequately with medication. At the time of writing, although a number of CBT manuals have been published (e.g. Fowler *et al.*, 1995), few professionals are trained in the technique. An additional difficulty in applying CBT is that users with the most intrusive psychotic symptoms have brief attention spans, requiring therapists to be flexible in their availability. We anticipate that the value of CBT will become clearer with further research and that training courses will be established to equip professionals with the essential skills. Meanwhile, it is worth reading one of the CBT manuals to gain an idea of the approach, with the caution that the techniques need to be applied in the context of a trusting relationship between therapist and user.

Cognitive coping strategies

I was having a full-fledged anxiety attack, and I said, 'I've had enough of this. If I'm going to die I'll just die. I don't care.' So I concentrated on my breathing and I said, 'I'm just going to get through this and I'm responsible for getting this woman home and I'm just going to do it.' So I did, and by the time we got home I was fine. So you learn to experience that even the worst mental health symptoms are not usually fatal. That's the part about getting older. You just sort of lose patience with the illness and you just say, 'I'm not going to pay any attention to it. I'm just going to let it happen if it happens, and I can deal with it.' So that's why I say my recovery is only half medication and half learning to handle it all.

5.3 Coping with paranoid delusions

A high proportion of people with paranoid delusions apply safety behaviours to counteract the perceived threat to themselves. Freeman and Garety (2004) studied 25 individuals with persecutory delusions. All used some type of safety behaviour: 92% avoided situations they perceived as dangerous, while 68% adopted strategies to use when in such a situation, e.g. protecting themselves by not opening the front door or decreasing their visibility by, for example, wearing a hat or cycling helmet or walking fast with eyes downcast. Almost two-thirds thought they achieved a degree of control over the situation.

A key aim of CBT is to construct alternative models of experiences that are acceptable to clients and not stigmatising. Early on, it is best to show care in the assessment phase, so that the logic of the delusion is not questioned. The therapist can focus on understanding how the belief developed rather than simply on its correctness or logical inconsistencies. In this way, a good understanding of the subjective experience is obtained while not risking loss of rapport. The ideal objective of therapy is the reduction of emotional distress via change in the degree of conviction in threat beliefs. Delusional beliefs are gradually weakened in the process of developing and assessing the alternative accounts of experience. Coping strategies can be used early in therapy to build trust in the relationship or to deal with high levels of emotional distress, before going on to evaluate beliefs.

5.4 Tackling negative symptoms

Although the meta-analyses by Davis *et al.* (2003) indicated that some atypical antipsychotics can reduce negative symptoms (see section 2.7), the effects are not great. It is necessary to apply other therapeutic approaches. Negative symptoms provoke critical attitudes in family carers, who do not appreciate that the symptoms are a product of the illness but instead attribute them to laziness, selfishness and other personality defects (Leff and Vaughn, 1985). Surprisingly, the same response is seen in professional carers for the same reason (Willetts and Leff, 1997). A number of controlled trials of psychoeducational family work have shown that it is possible to reduce critical attitudes of family carers after several months (e.g. Leff *et al.*, 1982). An educational programme based on family interventions has been developed and can produce similar changes of attitude towards users in staff working in long-stay wards (Willetts and Leff, 2003) and in community residences (Willetts and Leff, 1997). Interventions to change the attitudes of family and professional carers are an important prelude to gaining their cooperation in tackling the users' negative symptoms.

Reviving interests

It is helpful to start by exploring the user's experience of the problem. Some users disclaim interest in any activity, while others feel they lack the energy to attempt to do anything. For some years, the approach to a lack of interest was to reward users for activities approved by the hospital staff. The rewards tended to be small sums of money or cigarettes; this type of programme was called a token economy.

Such programmes were applied widely in the long-stay wards of psychiatric hospitals in the UK. The use of cigarettes as a reward is now ethically untenable, particularly in view of the excessive mortality of people with schizophrenia. Another common disadvantage of such behaviourally based programmes is the failure of any changes in behaviour to persist when the rewards are no longer forthcoming, for example after discharge to the community. The rewards that shape the behaviour of young children are approval from their parents and a sense of mastery over their environment. Approval from a teacher or therapist can still motivate an adult, and users whose illnesses have inculcated a feeling of inadequacy and helplessness can gain satisfaction from mastering a task if encouraged to rise to the challenge.

Rather than attempting to involve a user in a new interest, a better strategy is to explore the interests the user pursued before falling ill and attempt to revive those. Intersts might be playing ball games with other youngsters or enjoying art classes at school. Whatever the interest chosen to work on, the initial approach needs to be modest in scope, for instance watching a ball game on television together with a therapist so that a discussion of the match can be initiated during or after the game. Later on, the user could be encouraged to play a ball game with other users and members of staff. The psychosocial clubhouse, which we will learn more about in Chapter 13, can be very successful at involving unmotivated service-users in group activities. New members are assigned to work programmes that meet their interests most closely, for example the cooking unit. Although there is no strong pressure for the person to be actively involved right away, there is a group expectation that the person will begin to join in eventually.

Structuring the day

To start out with, I wrote everything down that I needed to do each day and I crossed it out as I went. That would make me get up in the morning because I had this list of things I had to do, to get started and get finished. It's like a grocery list. You know, you walk into a grocery store, you have a list, you cross out the things that you've got already. It helps you see something that you've done. The list is very helpful to me because you get to see everything that you crossed off. Then when you've finished, you can do whatever you want. That's the reward for getting through the day. Almost every day I do that.

Dealing with lack of energy

A user who is unable to undertake or complete a task may formulate the problem as a lack of energy, but it is likely to be compounded by low confidence and fear of failure, which are less easy to articulate. It is, therefore, essential to start with small, relatively undemanding tasks that are potentially achievable. Setting the targets too high will inevitably lead to failure and further erode the user's confidence. This is a common error made by family carers who are trying to activate the user. Family carers are invaluable allies for therapists attempting to alleviate negative symptoms, but in developed countries with a strong work ethic, expectations are often unrealistically high. Parents commonly expect the user to return to work or studies soon after recovering from an episode of psychosis, not realising that negative symptoms can endure for long periods of time. The situation is different in developing countries with traditional family structures. Relatives in extended families compared with those in nuclear families are more tolerant of users' minor behavioural abnormalities, allow them temporary withdrawal, have less expectation of feedback from the user, and are more successful in assisting the user to occupy their leisure time (El-Islam, 1982).

Family carers are usually willing to spend time and energy helping the user to achieve goals in the areas of self-care, domestic chores and leisure activities. However, it is necessary for therapists to work in conjunction with family carers to ensure that the tasks set are achievable, that the user is actively involved in choosing a task, and that the carers praise successful efforts and avoid criticism when the user fails to reach the agreed goal. When family carers persist with unrealistic expectations, it is an indication that they have not successfully mourned the losses resulting from their relative's illness. Engaging the carers in grief work (Miller, 1996) may enable them to move on to a more realistic view of their relative's capabilities.

Reducing social avoidance

We have indicated above that social withdrawal has the function of reducing the user's level of arousal, which is elevated by stressful social interactions. Allowing users time out from social situations is necessary in order to avoid a worsening of their psychosis, but shunning the company of others completely leads to inertia and a flourishing of psychotic symptoms unchecked by reality. Users who find the company of others unpleasantly arousing need to be helped to find ways of overcoming what amounts to a social phobia. Family members can help users tolerate a visit to the home by relatives or friends by discussing with them the possibility of leaving the company when they feel stressed and then returning a little later when they feel calmer. The user needs to be encouraged to prepare an excuse for his or her temporary absence from the room.

The environment of the psychosocial clubhouse (see Chapter 14) is designed to be not too intrusive or demanding. Members can sit quietly or work alone if they prefer, without excessive demands to interact with others. This allows members to gradually become more socially intimate at a speed that is not uncomfortable for them. The problem, however, is that even this environment can be too threatening for some people with marked fear of social contact, and these people will choose not to attend the programme initially. With gentle encouragement, however, they may begin to do so after a year or two.

Finding something to talk about

A common problem is not being able to talk to an acquaintance about something that is unconnected with illness or treatment. Social conversations tend to centre on jobs, relationships, interests and books read or films seen lately, all of which are likely to be in short supply for the average user. Some users need to learn that it is inappropriate to talk about their psychotic experiences to people other than family carers. A patient of one of us (JL), a young man who dressed smartly and fashionably and went to discos in the hope of finding a girlfriend, was unaware of this necessity. Within a few minutes of chatting up a girl, he would start telling her about the electronic chip in his knee through which he received messages.

A helpful approach to this problem is to run groups for users in which current affairs, recent films, sporting events and other topics of contemporary interest are discussed. As we learned, this was not a popular activity for very long-stay users (Morgan, 1979) (see section 4.6), since they had little or no opportunity to visit matches, cinemas and other places of entertainment that would furnish them with subjects to talk about. We hope that the transition to community care has increased the opportunities for users to spend their leisure time productively, although we have noted in the previous chapter that lack of finances imposes limits.

5.5 Social skills training

This approach developed out of behaviour therapy and was popular during the 1970s and 1980s. Since then it has fallen out of favour in the UK, although it is still alive and well in the USA. The need for many users with psychotic illness to improve their skills at interacting with others is clear. There is a common tendency to avoid eye contact and, among those with negative symptoms, to fail to smile or use brief verbal responses to encourage the other person to continue a dialogue. There may also be a failure to respond verbally to the other through slowness in thinking or distraction by intrusive thoughts or voices. Mueser *et al.* (1997b) point out that social competence requires the smooth integration of multiple component skills. This may be one of the reasons for the decline in interest in social skills, since our experience is that the individual components taught to a user are not convincingly absorbed into a seamless repertoire of social graces.

The other main deficiency that besets this form of therapy is evident from a meta-analysis of the relevant research conducted by Dilk and Bond (1996). These authors accessed publications and theses produced between 1970 and 1992 that evaluated the effectiveness of social skills training for adults with severe mental illness. They identified 39 studies that employed a control group and random assignment, all of which involved only inpatients. In most of these studies, the training period was brief, with a mean of 17.1 hours, and the follow-up period was three months or less. The overall effect size of the skills training was medium at the end of the course (0.40) but had increased to a large effect (0.56) by the follow-up. The authors conclude that behavioural skills training is effective for teaching inpatients interpersonal and assertiveness skills. However, few studies have examined whether training in a hospital setting generalises to social interactions in the community.

Mueser et al. (1997b) identified a handful of studies published after 1992 that involved users with schizophrenia who were living in the community. They acknowledged that the findings were not entirely consistent across studies, but they considered that, on balance, benefits were produced in social adjustment and symptom severity. They concluded that although the results were encouraging, further research was needed in order to clarify the value of social skills training for users in the community with schizophrenia and those with other diagnoses.

Despite the lack of firm evidence that what is learned in the training sessions generalises to everyday life situations, Mueser et al. (1997b) state that the wide availability of training modules and manuals 'has resulted in social skills training becoming one of the most commonly employed interventions for improving the social functioning of patients with SMI [severe mental illness]'. This assertion reveals a transatlantic divide: although it may represent practice in the USA, it certainly does not apply in the UK, where few services offer social skills training any more. The scepticism of UK practitioners may well be the unwarranted consequence of overselling social skills training in the early years and disappointment with the failure of acquired skills to generalise beyond the training setting. The answer to this deficiency could be to conduct training in real-life situations rather than in the clinic. The need for interventions to enhance users' abilities to interact socially is such a crucial prerequisite to social reintegration that an improved form of training should be a high priority.

5.6 Conclusions

Professionals need to be aware that their interventions sometimes may make the user's problems worse, as with institutional care. The same caveat applies to medication. The side effects of antipsychotic drugs on movement, facial expression and speed of thinking create barriers to social and occupational integration. Polypharmacy should be avoided, and dosage regimes should be kept to the minimum necessary to control symptoms but without inducing side effects. It is preferable to accept some persistence of delusions and hallucinations, which can now be tackled with non-pharmacological methods, than to burden the user with incapacitating side effects.

The development of a cognitive-behavioural approach to the control of delusions and hallucinations is promising, both in the acute phase of psychosis and for long-term symptoms that do not respond to medication. Its proper place in therapeutic regimes remains to be established, but it certainly deserves a trial when psychotic symptoms persist. However, the necessary therapeutic skills are not yet widely available.

Negative symptoms have been the target of cognitive-behavioural therapy, but with little demonstrable effect. However, novel antipsychotics do produce some improvement in negative symptoms, although the benefits are not large. Both professional and family carers become very critical of negative symptoms, with an adverse impact on the user. Critical attitudes of both types of carer can be modified by psychoeducational programmes, which are justified for many other reasons.

Apathy and lack of interest need to be tackled in order to assist users to integrate socially. It is more effective to build on previous interests than to introduce new ones. Group activities are helpful, as utilised in the clubhouse model. Family carers may have unrealistic expectations, which increase the user's burden. Carers need to be helped to develop realisable aspirations and encouraged to praise small advances by the user.

Some users are intolerant of social interaction and need to be introduced gently and patiently into social situations, allowing withdrawal when necessary. They often need help with finding something to talk about other than illness-related topics. Social skills training has fallen out of favour but may still be of use if undertaken in real-life situations.

Coping with stress

Getting too stressed, I get kind of crazy and I can't cope. So I really try to pace myself. I don't do anything during the week but go to work. If people ask me out I won't go over. All I want to do is do my job because my job pays me decent money. So I don't do anything during the week because it's too stressful. One day a month I call in and say I'm not coming to work, I'm not leaving my house, I'm going to take care of me. I can't do it any more. That's one day a month.

Dismantling psychiatric institutions

6.1 The legacy of the past

We have argued that the old-style psychiatric hospital perpetuates the stigma of psychiatric illness by virtue of its original isolation from residential areas, its exclusion from general medical services, and the custodial practices that came to characterise the care offered within its walls. The great programme of asylum building took place in the nineteenth century as a response to concern about the quality of care received by mentally ill people in private madhouses or confined in ordinary private households. The number of mental hospitals in the UK rose from nine in 1827 to 77 in 1900 (Carrier and Kendall, 1997). Initially spurred by humanitarian motives, the programme involved careful attention to the design of the hospitals, including the efficient circulation of air. The living spaces were large, with high ceilings and plenty of room for recreational activities. Airing courts were provided to enable the patients to exercise regularly.

It was the policy to site the hospitals in the countryside some miles from the nearest conurbation. This impeded visiting by relatives and friends, although in the case of Friern Barnet hospital, built some eight miles beyond the limit of Victorian London, the railway line was extended to reach the hospital. Unfortunately, once they were opened, the hospitals rapidly filled up with patients to well beyond their planned capacity. Friern Barnet hospital was built for 1000 patients and opened in 1851. The peak bed occupancy of 2400 was reached 100 years later. It was only in the 1980s when the beds had been reduced to their original planned number that the wisdom of the Victorian designers was revealed. Overcrowding had filled the recreational spaces with beds, and the sheer mass of patients made it impossible for the limited number of staff to give them individual attention. Instead, block treatment was instituted, with a uniform regime and loss of individuality. Patients were issued with hospital clothing, which was interchangeable, and no storage space was available for personal possessions.

Staff soon gave up on patients who failed to improve. Such patients were moved to 'back wards', where little therapeutic activity went on. Hence, it was common for patients admitted when young to spend the rest of their lives in the hospital. This helped to form the public view of the incurability of 'madness'. When the era of deinstitutionalisation dawned in the late 1940s and long-stay patients began to be considered for discharge, it was discovered that some women had been admitted decades before because they had become pregnant outside of marriage. They had never suffered from a psychiatric illness but had been admitted to extrude them from society. Evidently, asylums had been utilised to house people who were seen as a social embarrassment.

6.2 The past is still with us

The process of downsizing psychiatric hospitals has proceeded at varying rates in developed countries and has reached different stages. It is patchy throughout Europe, with the former Soviet bloc trailing the Western countries (Thornicroft and Rose, 2005). Even in Western Europe there are major differences between countries. In Great Britain the process began in the 1940s, but it did not get under way in Italy until the 1960s. Italy and Great Britain have now advanced furthest in Europe. Law 180 barred admission of any new patients to Italian psychiatric institutions beginning in 1978; instead, patients were to be admitted to small psychiatric units in general hospitals for acute care and subsequently treated in the community. The law mandated the ultimate closure of all the old institutions, and none is now open. England and Wales have closed the great majority of their psychiatric hospitals – over 115 of the 130 that were functioning in 1975. The USA has drastically reduced the number of psychiatric hospital beds but has closed a smaller proportion of hospitals than the UK. Most of the 50 states still have a functioning state psychiatric hospital, and a number of large Veterans Administration hospitals are in existence. Furthermore, physical restraint and seclusion are still in general use in US hospitals (Mattson and Sacks, 1983; Telintelo et al., 1983; Donat, 2003; Delaney and Fogg, 2005), whereas such methods are rarely resorted to in the UK or Italy. In Australia, one of the states has closed all its psychiatric hospitals, as has one province in Spain.

In other countries around the world, the psychiatric hospital still dominates the services. Until recently, the number of psychiatric beds in Japan was increasing steadily. Most of the Japanese psychiatric hospitals are privately owned by the psychiatrists who run them, and the state has little influence over the management of the hospitals. The Japanese government has offered financial inducements to psychiatrists to set up outpatient clinics and day hospitals, with little impact on the pattern of the services so far.

The authors have visited psychiatric hospitals in rural China, Indonesia, Macedonia, Mexico and Chile and found that the conditions under which patients live are depressing at best and dehumanising at worst. Overcrowding was so bad in one hospital in Hong Kong that patients had to climb over other patients' beds in order to reach their own beds. Working in a modern, community-based service, it is easy to forget the worst features of psychiatric institutions and to be unaware that in many places in the world they still project the image of the dangerous and incurable mad person.

6.3 Problems of decentralising a service

It is not a simple matter to relocate in the community the services provided within a psychiatric hospital. The asylums represented an extreme example of centralisation, with every service required being on a single site, conforming to Goffman's (1963) concept of the total institution. Patients lived, ate, worked and slept under the same roof. Spatial dispersal of these activities is necessary if a community service is not to reproduce the worst features of the asylums.

Deinstitutionalisation comprises three elements according to Bachrach (1976). Residents of psychiatric hospitals need to be resettled in community homes, wards in general hospitals should be provided for patients requiring admission, and a network of psychiatric and support services has to be developed. Together, these three elements need to reprovide all the useful functions of a psychiatric hospital, while curbing restrictions to the minimum possible and enabling the individual to participate fully in the social and economic life of the community.

What happened to industrial therapy?

The decentralisation involved in community services poses problems avoided by the centralised nature of the psychiatric hospital. Friern Barnet hospital, for example, ran an industrial therapy department attended daily by 120 users, some of whom commuted to the hospital from their homes in the community, where no equivalent facility existed. In the process of planning the closure of the hospital, it became evident that the industrial therapy unit could not be reproduced in the community because its users would be dispersed over too large an area, making travel to and from the unit unfeasible. One possible solution – splitting the department into subunits on scattered sites – was not practical because it relied heavily on contract work from large enterprises, necessitating quite a large workforce. The coordination of delivery, execution and collection of segments of the contract work from a number of sites was considered to be not viable economically.

In the event, a number of local sheltered workshops were established, each offering a diversity of work experiences. However, attendance at these facilities by the discharged long-stay users was poor. It emerged that when the users were free to choose what to do with their time, many preferred a drop-in centre, where there was no pressure to engage in structured activities. In response to this, a number of new drop-in centres were set up, mostly by voluntary agencies. It has to be emphasised that this long-stay population was elderly, with an average age of 55 years. The new population of users, both long-stay and short-stay, has different needs. The viability and usefulness of sheltered workshops for these groups of users will be addressed in Chapter 11.

Rehabilitation

There was little pressure to discharge patients from the old psychiatric hospitals. However, as the admission wards filled up, patients who had stayed for a number of months but were not ready for discharge were moved to intermediate-stay wards, where they took part in rehabilitation programmes. The staff running these programmes tended to focus on self-care and everyday living skills. As behavioural psychology developed, the principles of behaviour modification were introduced into the programmes. These included social skills training, which was designed to remedy the deficiencies many people with schizophrenia show in their social interactions.

Some patients responded well to these programmes while still in the hospital but failed to make the adjustment to community living. It became apparent that for people with schizophrenia, there was often a problem with generalising what they had learned in one situation (the hospital) to another (the community). The way to tackle this was to conduct the training in a situation that resembled as closely as possible the patient's eventual residence in the community. Optimally, the training should be provided in the community situation in which the patient was soon going to live. This led to the formation of community rehabilitation teams, which were based outside the hospital and took charge of patients who were being groomed for discharge.

The hospital-closure programmes in the UK took scant notice of the patients' needs for rehabilitation. There appeared to be an unspoken belief that the dismantling of the psychiatric institutions would put an end to chronic mental illness. Of course, this was unfounded, and the illusory optimism was shattered when it became evident that long-stay patients were accumulating on the psychiatric admission wards that had been opened in general hospitals. The problem increased in size, and surveys showed that around one-half of the new long-stay patients on admission wards could be discharged if there were adequate well-supported facilities in the community (Carey et al., 1993). Throughout the UK, in both urban and rural catchment areas, admission wards were operating well above 100% occupancy (Powell *et al.*, 1995) and dealing with this overload by transferring patients to private hospitals.

A national survey of rehabilitation facilities was conducted in England by Killaspy *et al.* (2006). A response rate of 89% of all National Health Service (NHS) trusts was achieved. Just over three-quarters of the trusts had short-term rehabilitation units with a length of stay up to 12 months. Each unit had a mean of 13 beds; this did not differ between urban and rural areas. Nearly all the units conducted a pre-admission assessment, and 42% had exclusion criteria. Most services had input from all members of a multidisciplinary team. Where there were both short-term and longer-term units, both tended to be covered by the same staff. Over half had a community rehabilitation team. The growth of these services has evidently occurred in recent years in response to the needs of the more disabled users. At the extreme end of the spectrum of disability are inpatients who are very difficult to discharge because of persistent severe psychotic symptoms and difficult behaviours, particularly aggression (Trieman and Leff, 1996). These individuals need long-term rehabilitation lasting several years (Leff and Szmidla, 2002), and few units can keep users for so long a period.

The alienating hospital environment

We were confined to an L-shaped ward with bedrooms, a small dining room, and a room where everybody smoked and some people played games like chess or Monopoly. There was a TV, but there was nothing at all to do with religion. I had to have somebody accompany me to mass, and they would wait until the last minute to say no one was available. So I think for six months at that hospital, I only went to mass maybe once or twice. There was no conversation. Everyone was treated like a dead body that you just pumped medication into. So I found this very disturbing. They put the person aside in the mental health system, through medication, but then they don't fill the person up with anything positive after that. The person is just left to flounder with television and small talk.

6.4 Problems with psychiatric admission wards

An important innovation of the deinstitutionalisation movement was the estab-lishment of psychiatric admission wards in general hospitals. A number of advantages of this policy were seen: a reduction in the stigma of mental illness, which would no longer be associated with the feared asylums, integration of a psychiatric service with the rest of medicine, ending the professional isolation of psychiatry, and accessibility of the patients to visitors, since the admission wards would be close to patients' homes. However, there were also disadvantages, which were not apparent at first.

Designing psychiatric admission wards

In the UK, the NHS is administered by central government, including the design of hospitals. The architects department of the NHS opted to use a modular design for all wards for reasons of economy. The assumption was that a basic ward unit could be utilised for any branch of medicine, surgery or obstetrics, with little modification. This thinking could not be applied to psychiatric acute care, since the bed here performs a different function from that in other medical disciplines. For psychiatric patients, the bed is not the place of treatment but merely somewhere to sleep. Treatment occurs in the other spaces on a ward – spaces that can be used for recreational and occupational activities, for socialisation and for individual and group treatments. This was understood by the architects of the psychiatric hospitals built in the nineteenth century but not by the modular designers of the twentieth century. As a result, many psychiatric admission wards in general hospitals are cramped and claustrophobic, with insufficient interview rooms and scant privacy for the patients.

One solution to this problem is to locate the psychiatric admission unit on the general hospital site but in a separate structure from the main building. The unit should be low-built, with no more than two floors, in order to reduce the danger to suicidal patients of jumping from a height. Ideally, there should be individual bedrooms in order to provide privacy and a place of refuge when the ward environment is very disturbed. Flexible spaces are needed for a variety of activities, and sufficient interview rooms are required for seeing patients and their relatives. There needs to be access to a secure garden that is screened from public gaze and provides sufficient space for aroused patients to walk about. Few units that incorporate these features exist in the UK.

6.5 Alternatives to hospital admission

The acute day hospital

Since the 1950s, a variety of innovative facilities have been developed in North America and Western Europe that are intended to avoid hospital admission for users experiencing relapses of their illnesses. These measures include day hospitals, crisis houses and crisis homes. The World's first psychiatric day hospital was opened in London by Joshua Beirer in the 1950s. Its purpose was to provide a place to which users could go to receive therapy, socialise and participate in recreational activities. Many more such hospitals followed and came to cater for two distinct types of user. One type was the user who had a long-standing psychiatric illness, who lived either independently or with family, and who needed somewhere to spend their weekdays taking part in the kind of activities offered by Beirer's pioneering facility. The other type was the user who had been under treatment in a psychiatric admission ward and was somewhat better but still needed ongoing treatment and care; for such users, the day hospital represented an intermediate stage between 24-hour hospital care and outpatient visits.

More recently, another type of day hospital has been instituted that aims to care for acutely ill users without admitting them to a ward. The acute day hospital, as it is known, accepts users who would otherwise be admitted to an inpatient ward. It cannot accept users who are admitted under sections of the UK Mental Health Act for legal reasons. Some other users are excluded from the acute day hospital because their clinicians consider them to be too seriously ill or because they are homeless. An evaluation of such a facility established in Manchester, UK, was conducted using a randomised controlled design (Creed et al., 1990). Two-thirds of the users allocated to day care were treated satisfactorily in the day hospital, a very similar proportion to that found in a similar study in the USA (Zwerling and Wilder, 1964). The Manchester team found that users living with relatives were more likely to be retained in day care when the families were visited by a dedicated community psychiatric nurse, who would instruct them in management of their relative.

Acute day hospitals are by no means available in every area of the UK, but examples exist in High Wycombe, Buckinghamshire, in North Kensington and East Ham, both districts of London, and in Dublin, Ireland. All of these operate from 9 a.m. to 5 p.m., seven days a week; some have slightly shorter opening hours at weekends. The small number of rigorous evaluations for this type of facility means that it is still regarded as being in an experimental stage. However, since the available evidence indicates that it is efficacious for a substantial proportion of users, and both users and their carers prefer this form of treatment to 24-hour hospital care, then there is good reason to provide this type of facility more widely.

Crisis houses

The rejection of institutional care for users with acute psychiatric illnesses has led to the innovative use of domestic environments by a few pioneering service providers. The use of open-door domestic settings avoids many of the restrictions of inpatient treatment and normalises the environment for people with mental illness. Such settings offer a number of benefits. They provide care that is much cheaper, less coercive and less alienating than hospital treatment, and they produce a different result than that of hospital treatment. People receiving services in a non-institutional setting are called upon to use their own inner resources. They must exercise a degree of self-control and accept responsibility for both their actions and the preservation of their living environment. Consequently, clients retain more of their self-respect, their skills and their sense of mastery. The domestic and non-coercive nature of the facility also makes human contact with the person in crisis easier than it is in hospital.

A good example of this kind of care is provided by Cedar House in Boulder, Colorado (Warner and Wollesen, 1995). Cedar House is a large home on a busy residential street, established in the 1980s. Users and staff like the facility because it is less confining, less coercive and less alienating than hospital admission wards. As a result, users make an effort to comply with house rules, and severely disturbed patients behave less aggressively than they would in hospital.

The staffing is equivalent to that of an acute psychiatric hospital ward, with nurses, a psychiatrist and mental health workers. The house offers all the usual psychiatric diagnostic and treatment services, except electroconvulsive therapy. As far as possible, it has the appearance of a middle-class home rather than a hospital. Residents and staff may bring their pets with them to the house. Staff and patients interact casually and share household duties. There are no locked doors, and residents come and go fairly freely after they have negotiated passes with their therapist. Nevertheless, many users are admitted involuntarily under the provisions of the state mental illness statute; they accept the restrictions because the alternative is hospital treatment, which virtually none prefers.

The people who cannot be treated in the house are those who are violent or threatening, who are so loud and agitated that they would make the house intolerable for other residents, or who are so confused that they cannot follow staff direction. The house cannot cope with people who repeatedly walk away or who are likely to abscond and as a result might harm themselves seriously. In practice, almost everyone with a psychotic depression, most people with an acute episode of schizophrenia and many people with mania can be treated in the facility. Many residents have a dual diagnosis of mental illness and substance abuse. Less than 5% need to be transferred to hospital. Cedar House has not entirely replaced locked hospital care, but it provides more than half of the acute inpatient treatment for the mental health centre's clients and could provide an even greater proportion if more beds of this type were available. It is striking that inpatient treatment at Cedar House costs half the daily rate in local psychiatric hospital wards. Similar acute treatment settings exist in Vancouver British Columbia, Washington DC, Trieste, Italy, and elsewhere.

A special type of crisis house that caters only for women has been set up in north London (Killaspy *et al.*, 2000). This house provides 12 places for women who would otherwise be considered for hospital admission. The women can have their children with them during their stay: the setting can accommodate up to four children over six months of age, with a maximum of two childeren per woman. The all-female staff consists of a project manager, 17 project workers, an administrative assistant and a cook. Excluded are women who need detoxification for substance abuse, women at risk of being violent and women who need constant supervision. The maximum stay target is 28 days, and the average length of stay during the first three years of operation was 19 days. Therapeutic work focuses on identifying and resolving the triggers to crisis using a systemic approach based on the model used in family therapy. The most common diagnosis is depression (53%), followed by schizophrenia (16%) and bipolar disorder (15%). The most frequent reason for admission is suicidal attempt or self-harm (47%), followed by relapse of psychosis (23%).

Crisis homes

An even more radical alternative was set up in Denver, Colorado, by Polak and colleagues during the 1970s and 1980s (Polak *et al.*, 1976). This consisted of a system of family sponsor homes for the care of users with acute psychiatric illnesses. The users were placed in a number of private homes, where they were helped through their crises by carefully screened and selected families. A mobile team of psychiatrists, nurses and other professionals provided treatment to the users placed in the sponsor homes. Surprisingly, this form of acute care proved to be suitable for the large majority of the catchment area's acute admissions. There is a historical precedent for this system. It was originally established in the town of Gheel in Belgium in the Middle Ages and replicated much later, in the mid twentieth century, by psychiatrist Tom Lambo. He established sponsor homes for acutely ill patients in the village of Aro in Nigeria. One of us (JL) visited Aro and asked the headman how Lambo had persuaded the villagers to accept the patients in their homes. The answer was that clean water and electricity were offered to the village in exchange for hosting the patients.

The crisis home system is no longer in operation in Denver, but it was used as a model for other agencies. In a review of the field, Stroul (1988) accessed information gathered from about 40 residential crisis programmes surveyed in a study by the US National Institute of Mental Health. She found that up to two-thirds of users thought to require hospitalisation were treated successfully in residential crisis settings. The length of stay in family-based crisis homes ranged from one night to 60 days, with an average of ten days to two weeks. A typical example of this type of care is provided by the Dane County Mental Health Centre in Madison, Wisconsin (Bennett, 1995). In that location, more than a dozen family homes provide care to a wide variety of people in crisis, most of whom would otherwise be in hospital. Nearly three-quarters of these clients suffer from acute psychotic illness and others are acutely suicidal. About 40% of the clients entering the programme are admitted from the community as an alternative to hospital care; 40% are patients in transition out of the hospital; and 20% are people whose clinical condition is not so severe as to require hospital care but who have housing problems or social crises. The average length of stay is only three days.

Violence by people admitted to crisis homes is almost never a problem. This is partly because of careful selection of appropriate clients and partly because clients feel privileged to be invited into another person's home and thus try to behave with the courtesy of house guests. For this reason, people with difficult personality disorders seem to behave better in crisis homes than they would in hospital wards. The crisis-home model has low fixed costs. Families are paid around US$85 for each day that a client is in residence. Consequently, such a programme can be established with a small number (four to six) of treatment places without significant loss of cost efficiency. For rural communities, the model has the advantage that the crisis homes can be dispersed widely, rather than located centrally like a hospital, making it possible to provide intensive treatment close to the client's home. To be effective, the treatment agency must sustain a high level of commitment to the success of the programme. Each foster-care family requires a substantial amount of support from a consistently available professional, and the patients placed in the home need intensive psychiatric treatment from a mobile team of professionals available 24 hours a day.

Given the stigma attached to psychiatric illnesses, one would anticipate that few people in the community would open up their homes to acutely ill people in this way. However, a programme of this type was launched in Boulder, Colorado, through a combination of newspaper articles and advertising. One hundred people called with an interest in the programme in the first month, and half a dozen homes were selected within a few weeks.

Stroul (1988) noted that neither crisis houses nor crisis homes were used widely and identified the problem as the obtaining of funds. The scarcity of these facilities has not changed substantially since then, prompting us to question why. In Britain, Australia and other countries with national mental health programmes that are still tied closely to a hospital base, it is necessary to close hospital beds in order to free up the necessary funding, a task that requires protracted bureaucratic negotiations. In the USA, where mental health programmes are often more independent of government, the task is more feasible; until now, however, health insurance mechanisms have not supported the use of crisis houses and crisis homes. US managed care providers are becoming aware, however, that non-hospital programmes offer cost/benefit advantages. Where per capita health-care schemes are being introduced in many states across the USA, we can expect to see hospital-alternative settings, with their opportunities for cost-saving, become used more frequently in preference to conventional care.

6.6 The location and size of staffed residences for users

Many users do not live with their families, either because there is no willing relative or because the user needs more specialised supervision from a psychiatric professional. Several issues are raised concerning the siting and size of staffed residences for users. We have discussed the issue of dispersing residences for users in order to avoid creating a psychiatric ghetto. However, there is a limit to the distances established between residences, dictated by the ease of travel between a residence and a facility for sheltered work, recreation or simply meeting friends. Ideally, such facilities should be within walking distance or accessible by a single form of public transport. In order to avoid reproducing the institutional features of psychiatric hospitals, staffed residences need to provide individual bedrooms and a comfortable communal living room in which residents can entertain visitors.

There is also the important consideration of the size and appearance of a staffed residence. If it is too capacious, it begins to resemble a mini-hospital in the community. When the number of residents reaches double figures, the building itself becomes conspicuous, standing out by virtue of its dimensions. Ideally, the exterior of a staffed residence should not mark it out as different from neighbouring dwellings. In some of the programmes in the UK, new buildings were planned to house discharged patients. These would inevitably have drawn the attention of neighbours, provoking those among them with prejudiced attitudes to raise objections or even mount campaigns against the users moving into the neighbourhood. Fortunately, the cost of new-build homes proved prohibitive and existing domestic housing was substituted.

Another consideration limiting the size of a group home is that a large number of ex-long-stay users with predominantly negative symptoms creates an inert mass that staff members struggle to activate. As argued earlier, it is advisable to select users so as to create a mix of socially active and isolated individuals, in order to facilitate the development of a cohesive network (Dayson, 1992). The staff in users' residences are not necessarily highly qualified. In fact, a survey of the staff in residences for long-stay patients discharged from Friern Barnet psychiatric hospital revealed that only one-half had received any form of psychiatric training (Senn *et al.*, 1997).

> **The alienating hospital environment**
>
> When I was in the hospital there were these sorts of things. In the morning if you wanted to get your toothbrush from the locked cabinet you had to go to the staff and say, 'Can I get my toothbrush?' Well the staff might say, 'Go away and come back in 15 minutes.' Or they would just ignore you. And I would think, 'How can I phrase this so this person will understand that I like to brush my teeth in the morning?' you know?

6.7 Changing staff attitudes

Although psychiatric hospitals were often built in the countryside, domestic housing for the staff and shops for staff and patients grew up around the perimeter. A family tradition of working in the hospital as nurses often became established, and in the older institutions several generations could have been employed in this manner. As a result, a nursing culture developed with a particularly custodial character. As deinstitutionalisation got under way, it became apparent that resistance to change was common among nursing personnel. One of us (JL) worked in a traditional mental hospital for eight years and was responsible for a group of 12 long-stay elderly male patients housed in the villa that formerly had been the residence of the physician superintendent of the hospital. In an attempt to normalise the environment, JL announced his intent to introduce female patients into the villa. The male nurse in charge fiercely resisted this change, protesting that it was immoral.

In order to avoid staff redundancies when closing hospital wards, it is customary to offer nursing staff posts in the newly established staffed community residences. In some countries, the nursing union may insist on this as a matter of policy. Although this appears fair and just, it entails the disadvantage that the staff carry with them the custodial culture of the hospital. Several studies have found high levels of expressed emotion (see Chapter 2, section 2.3) to characterise staff attitudes to users in community residences (Ball *et al.*, 1992; Snyder *et al.*, 1994; Willetts and Leff, 1997). Staff commonly direct criticism and hostility towards the users, although they rarely show overinvolvement. As with family carers, staff members' critical comments are focused mainly on the users' negative symptoms (Moore *et al.*, 1992). Despite their training, staff members, like the relatives, fail to recognise that negative symptoms are a product of a schizophrenic illness and not a mark of laziness or selfishness.

In view of these similarities with the attitudes of family carers, it was considered worth trying to change staff attitudes by offering them a modified programme of family work for schizophrenia (Kuipers *et al.*, 2002). In two consecutive studies, the training programme was given to staff in sheltered homes for discharged long-stay users (Willetts and Leff, 1997) and to staff working with 'difficult-to-place' patients in a psychiatric hospital scheduled for closure (Willetts and Leff, 2003). In the first study, the training course achieved a change in staff attitudes, which brought them closer to the users' viewpoint and equipped them with an increased range of coping strategies. The second course produced a significant increase in staff knowledge of schizophrenia and also the acquisition of strategies to achieve change. These two studies show that a relatively short course (nine to ten sessions) can alter the negative attitudes of staff members towards users and can extend their repertoire of effective strategies. This can help to activate users with negative symptoms and thus facilitate their engagement with life in the community.

6.8 Conclusions

Although psychiatric hospitals were introduced with the best of intentions and provided many useful functions, with the passage of time and the inexorable increase in the number of resident patients their value became subverted by custodial practices and an ethos of therapeutic pessimism. They have outlived their usefulness and have no place in a modern community-based service. Furthermore, they perpetuate the public stereotype of the incurable lunatic.

Replacing their valuable functions is not easy because of the decentralisation involved. Novel solutions need to be found for the provision of optimal facilities for rehabilitating users disabled by their illness; of staffed residences that ensure privacy and maximum autonomy; and of care during acute episodes of illness that deviates as little as possible from the normal conditions of life. Furthermore, the attitudes of staff members who worked in the previous system need to be changed to accord with the new philosophy of care. Pioneering services have been developed that fulfil all these requirements but still remain as scattered examples of the best practice. They have proved their worth and should become standard features of every psychiatric network of care.

Reducing fear and discrimination among the public

7.1 Using the mass media to influence public attitudes

We have discussed the bias of the media in selectively reporting violent incidents involving mentally ill people and in referring to such people in pejorative terms. This has an effect on the attitudes of the public towards psychiatric illnesses and service users. Given the ability of the mass media to reach entire populations of all ages, it is compelling to attempt to use them to instil positive attitudes about psychiatric illness. An early campaign in Canada by Cumming and Cumming (1957) targeting a local community was a dismal failure, the educators being rejected by the population. A similar attempt to change public attitudes in Northamptonshire, UK, was also ineffective (Gatherer and Reid, 1963). A national campaign was mounted by the UK Royal College of Psychiatrists, focusing on depression. Although a few significant positive changes occurred, they were disappointing given the effort invested in the campaign (Paykel et al., 1998). A subsequent attempt by the Royal College of Psychiatrists to reduce the stigma of a wide range of psychiatric disorders included a four-minute film that was screened before the main feature film in cinemas throughout the country. Once again, the impact on public attitudes was minimal.

The World Psychiatric Association (WPA) initiated a worldwide programme against the stigma of schizophrenia in 1996, which eventually involved 20 countries (Sartorius, 1997). The pilot site was in Calgary, a town in the Canadian province of Alberta. The pilot programme included an ambitious range of activities, which were evaluated carefully. An intensive educational campaign was launched using local radio. The effects of this endeavour were assessed by means of a before-and-after telephone survey of a random sample of the general population and by scrutinising the local newspapers and identifying articles featuring psychiatric illness. The population opinion survey revealed no positive changes in attitude towards or knowledge about mental illness. The newspaper articles were categorised as positive or negative and the total number of column inches of each category was calculated. By the end of the campaign, there was little overall change in the ratio of positive to negative articles. The campaigners explained the equivocal media response by the timing of several high-profile incidents involving mentally ill people. One was the break-in at the home of the Canadian premier. Others included the shooting of two police officers at the US Capitol and the arrest of the Unabomber, all of which occurred during the campaign. Although some of these incidents happened in the USA, they drew extensive press coverage in Canada. Such unpredictable events can cast their shadow over any media campaign and are difficult, if not impossible, to counteract.

The disappointing failure of large-scale media campaigns to change the attitudes of the public to psychiatric disorders lies partly in the resources available to fund them. Marketing campaigns mounted by commercial organisations continue for months or years and utilise radio, television, newspapers and hoardings. The cost is far beyond what a health service organisation could afford. Another explanation for the failure can be identified from the development of social marketing. Social marketing campaigns have been used successfully around the world in acquired immune deficiency syndrome (AIDS) prevention, smoking cessation and many other causes (Rogers, 1995). Effectiveness is increased by 'audience segmentation' – partitioning a mass audience into sub-audiences that are relatively homogeneous and devising appropriately targeted promotional strategies and messages (Rogers, 1996). In developing such campaigns, it is useful to conduct a needs assessment that gathers information about cultural beliefs and the media through which people could best learn about the topic. The needs assessment may incorporate focus groups, telephone surveys or information from opinion leaders. Specific objectives, audiences, messages and media are selected, and an action plan is drawn up. The messages and materials are pretested with audiences and revised. The plan is implemented and, with continuous monitoring of impact, constantly refined (Rogers, 1995).

7.2 Targeting high-school students

At the pilot site in Calgary, it was decided to select high-school students as one of the target groups. This choice was influenced not so much by the consideration that students would be a source of stigma but rather by their ready accessibility and the opportunity to influence the attitudes of a coming generation.

Gaining access to the students proved to be relatively easy. In meetings with school principals, the project members presented the stigma-reducing effort as an important component in diversity training and pointed out that mental illness is often neglected in health education in schools. Different methods of communicating the anti-stigma messages were utilised, since the impact of a social marketing campaign is increased if the target group receives the same message from a variety of sources (Smith, 2002). A teaching guide was prepared for the school staff, an art competition was held for the students to prepare anti-stigma materials, and people with psychiatric illness were recruited to speak to the students and answer questions.

This component of the programme in the pilot site was very effective in ameliorating the students' attitudes. The students' knowledge about schizophrenia and attitudes towards people with the illness were assessed before and after the programme. The proportion of students with a perfect knowledge score increased from 12% to 28%, and the proportion expressing no social distance between themselves and people with schizophrenia increased from 16% to 30%.

The success of this approach to high-school students led to replications in more than half the 20 countries participating in the WPA global campaign. In Boulder, Colorado, a speakers' bureau was constituted of a number of people with mental illness who were willing to talk to high-school students. An art competition was also organised with the support of the school principals and art teachers. Members of the speakers' bureau and a project coordinator with a visual arts background made presentations in art classes. The presenters announced a juried competition, with money prizes, for students to produce artwork dealing with stigma and mental illness. A public art show with an awards ceremony was mounted after each annual competition and the exhibit was displayed in participating high schools.

In Boulder, interior bus advertisements reach a predominantly younger audience and are free for public-service announcements. The Boulder project installed several anti-stigma bus advertisements, including one using student art with the statement, 'Sometimes those that are different are the most amazing'. Cinema patrons are also predominantly younger people. The Boulder project ran slides with three different anti-stigma messages among the advertisements preceding the main feature on 16 local cinema screens. One message read: 'Don't believe everything you see at the movies: mental illness does not equal violence'. Exit surveys revealed that 18% of cinema patrons recalled the content of at least one of the three messages displayed. Thus, during three months of displaying the slides, over 10000 people would have been able to recall one message two hours after seeing it. This results in a total cost of 36 cents per person-message, which compares very favourably with usual commercial media costs.

7.3 Targeting neighbours

The emptying of the psychiatric hospitals in developed countries necessitated the development of sheltered homes for thousands of discharged patients: very few patients could return to their family homes, because their relatives either had died or were unwilling to take on a caring role. In the reprovision for Friern Barnet and Claybury hospitals in London, only 4% of the long-stay patients were discharged to the care of their families. The great majority (78%) moved into staffed group homes (Trieman, 1997). Attempts to establish these homes some-times meet with opposition from neighbours in the area, the so-called 'not in my backyard' (NIMBY) response (Boydall *et al.*, 1989; Repper *et al.*, 1997). In an attempt to avoid this kind of opposition, service planners tend to keep the development of group homes as quiet as possible. Unfortunately, this strategy fails to take advantage of the considerable pool of goodwill in the community, revealed by public attitude surveys (Wolff *et al.*, 1996a). The alternative approach of educating the neighbourhood has much to recommend it but has been viewed by planning teams as risking stirring up opposition.

Wolff and colleagues (1996c) conducted an education programme for neigh-bours of a planned group home using an experimental paradigm. They studied two streets in south London, in each of which a staffed group home was to be opened for long-stay patients from the same psychiatric hospital. One street was chosen randomly for the education programme, while the other acted as a control. A survey was conducted in both streets before and after the programme, with assessments of knowledge of mental illness, attitudes towards mentally ill people and community care, and behavioural intentions towards those with a psychiatric illness. In addition, the social networks of the residents in the two group homes were determined before and two years after moving into the homes.

The materials for the education programme included a purpose-made video explaining the aims of moving patients into the community and featuring interviews with professional carers, local shopkeepers in another area with an established group home, and users. This was supplemented with information sheets on community care and psychiatric illnesses. A meeting for neighbours was held in a local church hall at which the video was shown and staff and a user were available for questioning. Copies of the video and information sheets were offered, by knocking on doors, to neighbours who had not come to the meeting. Social events, such as bring-and-buy sales and barbecues, were held in the group home, to which all neighbours were invited.

Compared with neighbours in the control street, those in the experimental street showed a small gain in knowledge and a significant reduction in fear of mentally ill people and the wish to exclude them from society. The neighbours in the experimental street were much more likely to know the names of the users, and to visit them, invite them in and count them as friends. This was confirmed by the assessment of the users' social networks. In the experimental area, five of the eight users had regular contact with neighbours compared with none of the six users in the control area. Two users in the experimental area each reported that they considered three of the neighbours to be friends.

Once again, targeting a specific group of people proved to be an effective way of reducing stigmatising attitudes and in this case led to a demonstrable outcome in terms of social inclusion of users. This experimental programme showed that it is possible to mobilise neighbours and translate their goodwill into friendly actions.

7.4 Working with family carers

Throughout the world, families are the principal carers of people with serious psychiatric illnesses, although the proportion of users who live with relatives varies from nearly 100% in traditional societies to less than half in Western cities. We have already discussed how many users do their utmost to conceal their illness through a justified fear of discrimination and rejection. Others, who are more confident and self-assured, risk disclosing the nature of their condition to friends and acquaintances. Family members respond similarly, many keeping their relative's illness a secret and withdrawing from social activities in order to avoid exposure. Although this is an understandable reaction, it only reinforces the silence surrounding psychiatric illness and does nothing to reduce ignorance and prejudice.

Speaking as a lone voice in a world perceived as hostile or indifferent requires considerable courage, but there is the possibility of joining together with others in the same situation, and that is much easier. Family carers have been establishing groups for many decades, but the degree to which these have developed into national organisations varies greatly between countries: in the USA the National Alliance for the Mentally Ill has thousands of members, but in many African countries, there is no such national association. In India, there are several strong local organisations, such as the Schizophrenia Research Foundation (SCARF) in Chennai (Madras), but these organisations have not amalgamated to form a national group. One of the hindrances to joining together can be differences in views about the nature and treatment of serious psychiatric illnesses. For example, in the UK the Schizophrenia Association of Great Britain has a strong ideological commitment to the dietary treatment of schizophrenia that is not shared by Rethink (formerly the National Schizophrenia Fellowship).

National organisations of family carers have the potential to exert considerable political clout on governments, and this can be used to lobby for changes in the law, improvements in services and increased expenditure on psychiatric illnesses. Politicians are more likely to respond to relatives, who represent many votes, than to professionals, who are seen to be acting out of self-interest.

Local groups offer many benefits to their members. Simply meeting others who are dealing with the same daily problems helps to reduce the sense of personal responsibility for the user's illness. Alleviating guilt in this way lowers the barrier to speaking out about the illness. Furthermore, carers learn from each other more effective ways of helping users cope with their symptoms and improve their daily living skills (Kuipers *et al.*, 2002, pp. 118–30).

Families that join a relatives' group also begin to form social bonds with others in the group and may share social activities with them outside of the formal meetings. This can benefit the users, who generally have small social networks. The reality is that many families are not willing to join such groups, particularly working-class families and ethnic minority families. Joining a group is itself an indication of openness about the term 'schizophrenia' and a willingness to discuss family problems with people who are, initially, strangers. For those who are reluctant to attend a group, working with the family on an individual basis can be very helpful to the users.

Work with a family begins with a short education programme that firmly asserts that families cannot 'cause' schizophrenia. It is essential for the professionals to gain the family's confidence, since many families will have had bad experiences of being blamed for their relative's illness. By being completely open about schizophrenia, the professionals model breaking the silence around the illness. They encourage parents who are overprotective of the user to socialise with people of their own age group, freeing the user to meet their own peers. However, serious psychiatric illnesses impair the individual's ability to make social contacts (see section 1.1) and help is required to overcome this problem. One possible source of assistance is a healthy sibling who might be willing to accompany the user to social activities or introduce him or her to their own social circle of age-appropriate friends. Siblings in this situation experience complex emotions about their ill brother or sister and need help with these from professionals before they are likely to take action (Kuipers *et al.*, 2002, pp. 97–8).

Family support

My husband's been very supportive to me. He was there for me each time when I had breakdowns, and he took care of me and took care of the financial end of it while I was in the hospital. I don't know what I'd do without him. My daughter's very supportive too. She calls me up quite often and talks to me and wants to know how I'm doing. We talk for a long time on the phone, sometimes almost three hours. And I talk to my mother every night, because if I don't call her she gets upset and worries about me.

Families are also a potential source of invaluable material for anti-stigma programmes. Real-life stories make more of an impact on the public than campaign slogans, and anecdotal experiences of being stigmatised either directly through association with serious psychiatric illness or indirectly through inadequate services and opportunities can be very moving. Only a minority of families are willing to expose themselves in this way, but they may be persuaded by stressing the power of their stories.

7.5 Working with the criminal justice system

We have cited evidence (section 3.5) that there has been no increase in violent acts by people with psychiatric illness over recent decades, despite the closure of many psychiatric hospitals, and that such violence is rare. Nevertheless, the linking in the media of mental illness with violence has had a powerful formative influence on the attitudes of the public, including police officers and criminal justice personnel. A mentally ill person who also has a criminal record is doubly disadvantaged in seeking acceptance by fellow citizens and employers. In some developing countries, and in rural parts of the USA with scarce psychiatric resources, jails are used to house people with serious psychiatric illness until they can be seen by a mental health professional, a practice that inevitably increases the stigma of these conditions.

Police and criminal justice officers are under-recognised partners in the management of mental illness. Police forces are extremely important local and national players in community services and, if used effectively, can contribute significantly to improving community awareness of mental health issues. People with mental health problems come into contact with the police both in everyday situations and in crises. Police officers bring people who are acutely disturbed at home or in public places into care or protective settings. Prison officers struggle to manage people with acute psychosis in environments totally unsuited to the task. Judges wrestle with the disposition of mentally ill offenders, and probation officers supervise mentally ill probationers without access to consultation regarding the person's capacity to respond to directives. And yet there are few examples of programmes that attempt to provide criminal justice personnel with the education necessary to perform these essential parts of their jobs. The teaching that is on offer focuses on the violence of psychiatrically disturbed people. This emphasis particularly affects inexperienced junior officers, who are then prone to use unnecessary force through an overreaction to a perceived threat of violence.

Police training

An example of what can be achieved by organising a training course for police officers is provided by the anti-stigma programme mounted in Boulder,

Colorado, as part of the WPA global programme. Mental health professionals, including one of the authors (RW), consumers and police officers collaborated in developing an eight-hour pilot training programme for seasoned officers and recruits in the county's largest city (population 100000). From the experience gained in this preliminary exercise, the project undertook the training of the entire police department in the county's second largest city (population 70000). To minimise the disruption of police services to the community, the training was delivered on six different occasions to a portion of the department's officers each time, at change of shift in the afternoon or evening before the officers went on duty. The training comprised two two-hour sessions on adult and child disorders, presented by psychiatrists, consumers and family members. The content included the features, course, treatment and outcome of psychotic disorders, myths about schizophrenia, suicide attempts, childhood disorders, and why people with psychosis should not be kept in jail. The classes discussed why people with borderline personality disorder are often not admitted to hospital. This topic is important if the training is to be successful, as police officers everywhere are likely to complain about bringing in a person for evaluation after a suicide attempt, only to learn later, as commonly phrased, 'They got home before I did!'

Pre-/post-testing of the officers revealed no change in attitudes towards people with psychosis but a 48% improvement in knowledge scores. The proportion of officers holding inaccurate beliefs about the causes of schizophrenia fell from 24% to 3%. However, the proportion holding a mistaken belief about the usual behaviour of people with schizophrenia only reduced from 82% to 71%. After training, 71% of officers still believed one or more of the following statements: people with schizophrenia are (i) always irrational, (ii) much more likely to be violent than the average person or (iii) usually unable to make life decisions. We realised subsequently that police encounters with people with psychosis nearly always occur when the person is acutely disturbed, and officers have little opportunity to meet people with schizophrenia who are working, in stable relationships or rarely need admission to hospital. We concluded that police training must intensively expose officers to people who have recovered from psychosis if it is to effect attitudinal change. Subsequent police training sessions in Boulder county ranging from four to seven hours in duration have achieved modest improvements in attitudes and substantial knowledge gains.

Judges, attorneys and probation officers

In the Boulder campaign, psychiatrists, people with mental illness and family members provided three training sessions on adult disorders and one session on child disorders to judges, attorneys and probation officers. Nearly all the county judges attended. An assessment of the judges' understanding before and after the training revealed that their knowledge of schizophrenia improved from 47% to 74% accuracy; some reported immediate changes in sentencing practice. Subsequently, the judges requested two more training sessions on juvenile disorders.

Another approach that avoids the criminalisation of psychiatrically ill people has been introduced in several services in the UK; this is known as a court diversion scheme. Its aim is the transfer of people with mental disorders from the criminal justice system to an appropriate psychiatric service if indicated. One such scheme in southern England operates during normal office hours Monday to Friday, and is led by community forensic nursing staff (Kingham and Corfe, 2005). During a three-year period, 1830 referrals were made to the scheme, 40% of which came from the police. A study of these referrals found that the majority (71%) were people detained in police custody who had been recently arrested; 8% were in prison, having been remanded by the court in custody. The majority (83%) of those referred were assessed by a community forensic nurse; 16% were seen by a doctor. The commonest diagnosis was drug misuse (19%), followed by alcohol misuse (12%) and schizophrenia (11%). A recommendation by the nurse or doctor for diversion or liaison was made in 47% of cases, of which the court rejected only 4%. The majority of people assessed in this scheme were seen soon after their arrest and before their appearance in court. This differs from other diversion schemes that operate solely within a court, for example in the city of Glasgow (White *et al.*, 2002).

7.6 Coordinating activities for social inclusion of mentally ill people

The programmes described above involve activities directed at many different sections of the community. An effective way of organising and coordinating some or all of these activities is to set up an action committee.

Establishing a local action committee

An action committee brings together members of the local community who have a strong interest in facilitating the social and occupational inclusion of people with psychiatric illnesses. Committee members should include representatives of potential programme target groups, although these will not be known when the action committee is formed. The initial planning group, therefore, should select committee members from walks of life that are likely to become target groups, such as police officers, employers and clerics, and add members later as needed. Some of the most valuable members of the action committee will be users and family members, who understand first-hand the experience of discrimination.

Action committee members must be willing to devote substantial time to the programme, as most of the work will be accomplished by their volunteer efforts.

It is valuable to include prominent citizens (e.g. legislators) on the committee. When requesting a meeting with, say, the editorial board of the local newspaper, the inclusion of someone whose name is well-known increases the impact. Prominent individuals may have less time to commit and can, therefore, be given affiliate status.

An action committee should comprise 10 to 20 members: neither so small as to burden members with too much work nor so big as to be unwieldy. A large group can split into taskforces to refine action plans for different target groups. Action committees commonly meet monthly, distributing minutes and an agenda at each meeting.

Selecting target groups

In deciding on the groups to target, it is helpful to conduct a survey of local users, family members and others to determine where stigma and exclusion are seen to be prevalent (e.g. in emergency rooms, by employers). Using this information, the action committee should select a manageable number (probably no more than three) of target groups. Target groups should be homogeneous and accessible. Landlords, for example, are not an accessible group, since they do not meet as a group or use a common media outlet. Employers are more accessible because the committee can identify the largest local employers and target their human-resource departments. Police officers are an accessible group, as they receive regular in-service training.

Setting up a user speakers' bureau

A speakers' bureau is valuable for addressing students, police officers and other groups. Such a bureau often comprises people who have experienced mental illness, family members, and a mental health professional whose function is to answer factual questions (e.g. 'What causes schizophrenia?'). Research on public attitudes suggests that personal contact with someone who has a psychiatric illness ameliorates negative stereotypes (Link and Cullen, 1986; Penn *et al.*, 1994). However, users are vulnerable people and can react to the stress of public speaking by experiencing an increase in symptoms shortly after the event. To minimise this possibility, users with good stress tolerance should be selected. They should be introduced gradually to the speaking experience by first observing and then speaking briefly, until they can participate fully without stress. Speakers should be debriefed after each presentation in order to learn what they found stressful. Several speakers should be trained so that the demand on any single individual is not too great.

User speakers demonstrate the reality of recovery, generating optimism and compassion. A study conducted in Innsbruck, Austria (Meise *et al.*, 2001), revealed that high-school students addressed by a psychiatrist and a consumer reported significant changes in social distance attitudes, while those who were addressed by a psychiatrist and a social worker did not. Users can talk about discrimination in employment, housing and law enforcement, but they should try to avoid generating defensiveness in the audience.

The speakers' bureau coordinator can be a user, family member or enthusiastic citizen. He or she should maintain a diary of engagements, select speakers for each event, debrief speakers afterwards and ask the host to provide an assessment. The speakers and the coordinator commonly receive remuneration. A successful speakers' bureau, such as the Partnership Program operated by the Calgary branch of the Schizophrenia Society, will develop a strong sense of shared mission that is nurtured through regular meetings.

7.7 Conclusions

The first attempts to change public attitudes by working with entire communities failed, and led to an understanding that programmes operating on a local level were more likely to succeed. A number of local initiatives have produced encouraging findings by targeting specific groups, such as the neighbours of a staffed group home, high-school students and the police. Programmes aimed at a variety of target groups have been established under the WPA Global Programme to Reduce Stigma and Discrimination because of Schizophrenia. Experience in running these programmes has demonstrated the importance of setting up local action committees comprising users, family members, public figures and members of the target groups. A speakers' bureau made up of users, family members and a psychiatric professional is a valuable resource for initiatives with the target groups.

This is a relatively new field of social intervention and investigation, and there is much more to be learned about the most effective and efficient methods of achieving change. The WPA programme, by involving 20 countries, has provided a unique opportunity to compare different approaches to reducing stigmatising attitudes and facilitating integration of people with psychiatric illnesses. It will also generate information about the modifications needed to adapt programmes to suit local cultures.

Tackling self-stigmatisation

8.1 Normalising unusual experiences

We have discussed the response of users to discrimination and stigmatising attitudes (section 3.7). A small minority of users speak out about their experiences and act as champions for their cause. The great majority, however, react by withdrawal and concealment, isolating themselves from possible sources of help. The effect of isolation is to compound the user's sense of being uniquely abnormal. In fact, the hallucinatory experiences of users suffering from psychoses are by no means unique. It has been known for many decades that around one half of people who have lost a loved one see, hear or feel the deceased person, sometimes for years after the loss (Rees, 1971). Rees pointed out that bereaved people are very reluctant to talk about these experiences for fear of being thought 'mad', and none of his informants had revealed them to a doctor. More recently, surveys of the general population enquiring about unusual perceptual experiences and beliefs have found that between 5% and 18% acknowledge isolated psychotic experiences that do not seem to bother them (van Os *et al.*, 2000; Johns *et al.*, 2004). In support of these findings, an Internet survey of over 1000 members of the public that was focused on paranoia revealed that between 10% and 20% of the respondents held paranoid ideation with strong conviction and significant distress (Freeman *et al.*, 2005).

There remain many traditional cultures where a belief in the existence of a spirit world is held firmly by the majority of the population. In such cultures, a person reporting that he or she heard the voice of an ancestor would be considered fortunate rather than ill; as a consequence, people who talk to themselves or to imaginary voices are not taken to traditional healers (Cheetham and Cheetham, 1976). Imparting the above information to a user who is hearing voices or holding unusual beliefs would likely reduce the unpleasant feeling of being an unacceptable outsider. The same benefit could be achieved by joining with other people who have psychotic experiences and sharing these. That is one of the main purposes of Hearing Voices groups. A pioneer in establishing this kind of group was Marius Romme in the Netherlands (Romme and Escher, 2000). In the summer of 2000, while in the UK, Romme launched the Hearing Voices Network. In his opening speech he stated:

Hearing voices in itself is not a symptom of an illness, but is apparent in 2–3% of the population ... There are in our society more people hearing voices who never became psychiatric patients than there are people who hear voices and become psychiatric patients . . . The difference between patients hearing voices and non-patients hearing voices is their relationship with the voices. Those who never became patients accepted their voices and used them as advisers . . . In these groups of voice hearers, people can learn from each other about coping with their voices and they can support each other in the battle to stop being discriminated against.

Following this launch, a number of voluntary organisations, such as Mind, set up similar self-help groups. There are now over 80 of these groups in the UK, as well as many in other European countries. In addition to diminishing users' sense of isolation and normalising their experiences, the groups provide a forum for the sharing of methods of coping with persecutory voices, enabling group members to learn from each other, as Romme suggests.

The authors of the internet survey of paranoid ideation (Freeman *et al.*, 2005) made the following clinical recommendations based on their findings:

Interventions may be more effective if they include recognition of the ubiquity of suspiciousness; encourage talking about such experiences with others; improve self-esteem; help people in negotiating relationships with others; and encourage detachment and feelings of control over the situation.

8.2 Working with the family

We have seen that users can encounter discrimination from their own family members and that relatives can maintain a silence about the user's illness. This can be tackled during psychoeducational sessions with the family by encouraging the user to describe their experiences. An atmosphere conducive to disclosure is created by therapists being open about the diagnosis of schizophrenia and its symptoms from the start. Once the user begins to talk about their hallucinations or delusions, therapists should emphasise that these are common experiences of people with mental illnesses. Sometimes, after a user has spoken about a particular experience, a genetically related family member may be prompted to disclose that they had something similar previously for which they never sought help. Relatives can experience transient episodes of psychosis as a manifestation of schizophrenia spectrum disorder. In one family with which JL worked, the user described believing that passengers on public transport moved away from her because she smelled bad. Following this, her mother reported that some years previously, she used to feel that there was a stranger hiding in the house whenever she entered it. She did not seek help for this frightening experience and after some time it faded. Such disclosures by family members can help to reduce the sense of alienation and rejection that many users feel.

8.3 Cognitive therapy for low self-esteem

Cognitive therapy was developed initially for the treatment of depression and focused on the user's self-esteem, which was invariably low and believed to be the root cause of depressive symptoms (Beck, 1976). Depression is a common component of schizophrenic illnesses and does not always resolve when the psychotic symptoms respond to treatment (Leff *et al.*, 1988). There is a substantial body of evidence for the efficacy of cognitive therapy in treating depression and the associated low self-esteem. Unfortunately, the research on cognitive-behavioural approaches to schizophrenia has rarely included measures of users' self-esteem.

However, one group pioneered an intervention designed to improve self-esteem in people with schizophrenia. Lecomte, Cyr and colleagues (1999) developed a module that addresses five areas: security, identity, belonging, purpose and competence. They evaluated the efficacy of their intervention in a controlled trial in which patients with schizophrenia were randomised to either a control stream or an experimental stream. The experimental intervention was given by two clinical psychologists to groups of eight participants. The Rosenberg Self-Esteem Scale was used as a measure but failed to show any effect of the intervention. The module was aimed not at the acquisition of specific behavioural skills but rather at the development of knowledge about oneself, including one's qualities and strengths.

A different approach to therapy was taken by Hall and Tarrier (2003). Their intervention merits detailed description, as it was shown to be efficacious in a randomised controlled trial. The subjects were inpatients on an acute unit who suffered from chronic schizophrenia. Those randomised to the experimental group received seven sessions of therapy delivered weekly. Patients were asked to produce a list of ten positive qualities or statements (two per session) that they considered pertained to themselves. They were then asked to rate the strength of their belief that they possessed this quality on a 0–100 scale. The therapist went through the list with the patient, and for each positive quality the patient was asked to give as many actual examples as they could of them displaying this quality. They were then set a homework exercise to monitor their behaviour over the next week and record specific evidence to support positive qualities in their actions. Examples of such evidence include 'Even when I walk down the street, I meet about half a dozen friends' and 'I'd do without to see my daughter happy.'

The experimental and control patients were compared initially, immediately following the intervention for the experimental group, and at a three-month follow-up. There was a significantly greater increase in self-esteem, measured by the Robson Self-Concept Questionnaire, for the experimental patients after treatment and at follow-up. The experimental patients also showed significantly greater improvement than the control patients in positive and negative symptoms and in social functioning. Since symptoms and social functioning were not addressed in the intervention, the findings suggest that improvement in self-esteem has an influence on these aspects of users' illness and behaviour. The beneficial effect on social functioning is particularly important in terms of social integration.

The main problem with this study was the attrition of the original sample. As many as 61% of eligible patients declined to participate, and others dropped out during the course of the study, leaving only ten experimental patients and eight control patients in the three-month follow-up. Despite these small numbers, significant differences emerged between the groups, suggesting a powerful effect of the intervention. It is necessary to attempt to replicate this study with a much larger sample, paying attention to the problems of stimulating users' interest in taking part.

Family attitudes and self-esteem

Tarrier's group has examined the relationship between users' self-esteem and the attitudes of family carers (Barrowclough *et al.*, 2003). They studied 59 users with schizophrenia of less than three years' duration and measured self-esteem with the Rosenberg Scale and also the Self Evaluation and Social Support (SESS) interview of Andrews and Brown (1991). The SESS generates scores on both negative and positive self-esteem, which are not necessarily related inversely. The emotional responses of the key family carer were assessed with the Camberwell Family Interview.

On the Rosenberg Scale, the users scored significantly lower than normal people. On the SESS, the users had moderately high negative self-evaluation and moderately good positive self-evaluation. A significant correlation was found between negative self-evaluation and a total score on symptoms. This was relatively strong for both delusions and hallucinations. These researchers found that the more critical comments the relatives made, the higher was the user's score on negative self-evaluation. Hostility expressed by relatives was linked with a low positive evaluation of self and greater negative evaluation of role performance.

The authors interpret these findings as showing that criticism and hostility from family carers reduce users' positive regard for themselves and increase their negative self-evaluation. These in turn intensify delusions and hallucinations. If this interpretation is correct, then working with the carers to reduce criticism and hostility should improve users' self-esteem. Family work has been shown to be effective in reducing the negative attitudes of carers (Kuipers *et al.*, 2002) and should be considered as an approach to raising self-esteem.

Insight and self-esteem

We saw earlier (section 3.7) that users with a first episode of psychosis who refused to accept that they had a mental illness had higher self-esteem than those who showed good insight (Morgan, 2003). This research supports the findings of Doherty (1976) and a partial replication of Doherty's results by Warner and colleagues (1989). This group tested the hypothesis that labelling and stereotyping are so damaging that patients who accept that they are mentally ill have a worse outcome than those who deny it. They studied 54 people with psychosis living in the community in Boulder, Colorado. Their results provided some support for the hypothesis but did not fully confirm Doherty's findings. Patients who accepted that they were mentally ill had lower self-esteem and lacked a sense of control over their lives. Those who experienced mental illness as most stigmatising had the lowest self-esteem and the weakest sense of mastery. Neither rejecting the label of mental illness nor accepting it, by itself, leads to good outcome. Users can benefit from accepting they are ill only if they also have a sense of control over their lives. Such users are few and far between, however, since a consequence of accepting the illness label is a loss of sense of mastery. This is the catch-22 of being mentally ill in Western society: in the process of gaining insight, one loses the very psychological strength that is necessary for recovery.

A conclusion we can draw from this research is that it is equally important for therapists to assist patients in developing a sense of mastery as it is to help them find insight into their illness. However, this is not what conventional treatment programmes do. Ordinarily, a good deal more effort is expended on persuading patients that they are ill than on finding ways to put them in charge of their illnesses.

8.4 Creative activities

The question of whether creative people are more prone to mental illness has long been debated in scientific literature, with the examples of Vincent van Gogh, who committed suicide, and Richard Dadd, who killed his father, often being cited. Art therapy was an integral part of treatment in the more enlightened psychiatric hospitals, but it has suffered a steep decline with the transition to community-based services. Nevertheless, encouraging users to express themselves and their experiences in a medium of their choice offers undeniable benefits, even though its value has rarely been the subject of scientific research.

The opportunity to translate frightening or exhilarating experiences into a two- or three-dimensional form that can be shared with others and discussed can reduce some of the immediacy and intensity of the experiences. By objectifying their experiences, users gain a degree of distance from them. Furthermore, despite, or perhaps because of, the naivety brought to the works by untutored people, such products have an eye-catching appeal. Indeed, art collectors have labelled the work of people with mental illness 'outsider art' and 'art brut'. These terms have unfortunate connotations, but they have had the effect of rendering such works desirable acquisitions and some have been bought for large sums. The work of people with mental illness has also been presented in prestigious exhibitions in public and private galleries.

Creative activity

I do art work. I write. It's a release of tension. I write 'Dear God' letters. I just recently did some paintings. I gave one to a fellow artist in the church and she gave me a flower arrangement in return. Now that it's fall, I'm getting inspired with the gold and the oranges and the reds.

A pharmaceutical company, Janssen, mounted an art competition for people with schizophrenia two years running. The entries were generally of a high standard, and the 12 winning entries were featured in a published calendar. The winners and a number of other works submitted were displayed in an exhibition in a private gallery. The valorisation of artwork produced by people with serious mental illness must have an effect in raising the self-esteem of the artists, but it could also boost the sense of worth of all users. An enquiry by Mind (1999) into users' experience of discrimination and ways of promoting social inclusion quotes evidence from a witness: 'We believe the arts can play a major role in developing excluded groups' confidence and ability to take an active role in their communities, and for the work they do through the arts to be a major tool in breaking down individuals' or communities' prejudice and preconceptions.' Another witness, Francoise Matarasso of Comedia, stated:

There are many examples of arts in mental health work – for example the involvement of mental health service users by Nottingham Museum Service in education and outreach work which has been long and patient and very successful. The people involved benefit in terms of personal confidence, by being included in activities that aren't presented as therapeutic, i.e. only targeted at them as service users. Then there is a significant impact on their social lives and confidence.

Theatre and poetry are other media to which users have contributed. A group in Calgary, Canada, wrote a play about a user with schizophrenia who heard voices. Different users acted the parts of the voices, while one user played a somewhat caricatured psychiatrist. The play, *Starry, Starry Night*, was very successful and toured several Canadian towns. The production helped to reduce stigma, and the actors gained the confidence to appear in front of audiences. The WPA programme against the stigma of schizophrenia recommends that:

several if not all members acquaint themselves with every role in the play so that roles become interchangeable. The more they play the different roles the more they feel at ease in their participation. This assists them at the end of the play when they invite the audience to ask questions. In general, patients report a feeling of empowerment and of accomplishment for their acting and they learn to decide when they can participate or abstain.

Newssheets produced by voluntary organisations and some national journals, such as *Schizophrenia Bulletin*, regularly publish poems by users. Poetry appears to provide a medium that is conducive to the expression of unusual states of mind. Some users' poetry is trite, but seeing it in print must give the authors a sense of achievement. One of us (JL) looked after a user whose main symptom of schizophrenia was thought disorder. He started to write poetry that reflected his disordered thinking. However, a local group of poets was impressed by his poetry, taking it for an avant-garde creation, and encouraged him to give readings to the group. As the user's condition improved, his poetry became more coherent and eventually was published in a national magazine.

8.5 The rise of the user movement

We have seen that when users who hear voices meet together regularly, they all benefit from a sense of belonging to a group of like-minded people. Such groups engender a feeling of solidarity, but by their nature they remain on the periphery of society. In order to exert political influence, users need to form national organisations with clearly stated aims and objectives and a large membership. Only then will they have any chance of being listened to by governments and to have at least some of their demands met. Since the 1980s, user organisations have been established in a number of developed countries and some have become national in status. In the UK, Mind is a national users' organisation that receives a sizeable annual grant from the government. In fact, its grant is several times larger than that given to the National Schizophrenia Fellowship (now called Rethink), which mainly represents relatives. In the USA the two most prominent organisations of service users are the National Mental Health Consumer Association and the National Alliance for Mental Patients, but there are many others, several of which operate frequently used websites, such as the National Empowerment Center (www.power2u.org) and the National Mental Health Consumers' Self-Help Clearinghouse (www.mhselfhelp.org).

Changes in the doctor–patient relationship

The rise of the user movement needs to be viewed in the context of large-scale societal changes affecting the relationship between professionals and their clients. Since the Second World War, there has been a gradual flattening of the hierarchy of the medical profession. This hierarchy used to have the form of a steep pyramid, with the specialist physician, surgeon or obstetrician at the summit and the patients at the lowest level. Information flowed upwards, and orders were transmitted downwards. At the beginning of his medical training, one of us (JL) would regularly encounter patients with extensive surgical scars who had no idea what operations had been performed on them. This offers a dramatic contrast with the situation today, where patients have complete access to their medical notes, including the results of all investigations. The balance of power has largely been equalised.

Users of psychiatric services have benefited from these societal shifts in the balance of power, although the unique necessity in psychiatry to compel some users to be admitted to hospital and receive treatment against their will leaves considerable power in professional hands. However, in the UK, psychiatric users serve on ethical committees and collaborate with scientists in the design of research studies. In the USA, users are often members of the governing boards and advisory boards of their service agencies and serve on the executive committees and quality-improvement committees of the same agencies, These responsibilities inevitably boost the self-confidence of users and enable them to feel that their contributions are valued. The increasing confidence of users can lead to them challenging the psychiatric system and sometimes organising anti-psychiatry demonstrations. However wrong-headed this may seem to the professionals, it is vital to respond rationally and to recognise that no system is perfect and that users' complaints must be taken seriously.

8.6 Promoting social inclusion

Although undoubtedly users benefit from gaining greater confidence and increasing their self-esteem, their integration into society requires a reciprocal response from other citizens. The prejudices and stereotyped ideas held by the public mean that a positive response to social overtures from users cannot be taken for granted. However, there are organisations in the community that can facilitate the social inclusion of users, including social clubs run by religious groups, befriending schemes and adult education classes.

Religious groups

In Ethiopia, the Coptic Christian churches are centres of healing, carried out by priests. Among the many people who come to be healed are those with serious mental illnesses. If they do not respond rapidly to the healing rituals, they are allowed to stay on in the compound of the church (Giel *et al.*, 1968). It is evident that in the Coptic healing centres, mental illnesses are integrated with all other kinds of sickness. Some Western Christian churches, particularly the evangelical sects, also undertake healing. However, there is a reluctance to attempt to heal people with psychotic illnesses.

Churches often run social clubs that all are welcome to attend. One would expect that people with mental illness would also be welcomed at such clubs, giving them the opportunity to socialise with ordinary members of the public, but this is not always the case.

Church support

I went back to Christ and I got a lot of support from my church. I had members of my church come visit me about once or twice a month, sometimes three times. And I went to church weekly. They have wonderful people there. It is a brotherhood and a support system and you can pick up the phone and call just about any church member and ask them for help and they'll help you.

Adult education classes

Like church social clubs, adult education classes are open to anyone. They also provide the opportunity to mingle with people outside the sphere of mental illness. Classes have the advantage of catering to a wide range of interests and abilities. There is no pressure to prove oneself in examinations or to reach a high level of achievement. Furthermore, one may attend for a single term, a full year or several years. The fees for attendance are usually not high, and concessions are available for unwaged people. Classes are particularly valuable in providing a structure to the week for people without employment and act as places at which to make informal social contacts.

Befriending schemes

We have already noted the difficulty people with serious mental illnesses experience in making new friends, which is partly responsible for the small size of their social networks. As a result, their social lives are often restricted to immediate family. Furthermore, younger users may be forced to spend much of their leisure time inappropriately with the older generation of family carers. This problem has been addressed by setting up befriender schemes. Such schemes are usually run by voluntary organisations, which recruit ordinary citizens to act as befrienders to people with serious mental illnesses. Befrienders need to be selected carefully to match individual users' preferences and needs. Befrienders should also be given some instruction about serious mental illnesses and what to expect from their clients. For example, befrienders need to be warned that the user may not smile or show much warmth, since the illness can restrict the expression of feelings. Simply having a non-judgemental person to talk to about everyday matters can be highly appreciated by users.

Social integration

I was scared of life, scared of people. I just wanted to isolate myself and get rid of my life. Going to classes and daily Mass I slowly replaced the sorrow and negativity with positive things in life. That's what most people live on. I could see that by keeping myself busy I was doing myself a favour. I signed up for some classes at the university and I liked that very much. It was social; you got to meet happy people; they were nicely dressed and you got to talk with them, find out a little bit about them, which was interesting. Everybody was different and it was fun. I felt that giving my intellect a structure was helpful – it gave me a discipline. I had to accomplish something. It was helpful because my mind had become useless as if it could be thrown out because I hadn't done anything with it. The structure for using my intellect and then the social activity to build up my positive affirmation of life – those things were very helpful.

I was always very isolated and at least now I am talking to people. Sometimes I go to the movie with them, sometimes I have lunch with them. I'm not very social and I don't know if I would like to be. But the social thing is very important for someone who has an illness. You need to not feel alone in this world because it makes you afraid and you need to feel loved.

8.7 Conclusions

The natural response of family carers to the person who reveals their unusual experiences is to deny the reality of the experiences. The individual may then begin to doubt their own sanity, and this is likely to be reinforced by professionals with whom they come into contact. The resulting lowering of self-esteem is damaging to the user's confidence and can lead to progressive isolation from social support networks. Joining groups of other voice-hearers combats isolation and normalises unusual experiences. Promotion by professionals of open discussion of the user's experiences with their family has a similar effect.

Low self-esteem can be tackled directly by a cognitive-behavioural approach. This type of intervention for people with psychoses is still in its infancy, but there are encouraging indications that if it is successful in boosting users' self-esteem, then there may be added benefits in the improvement of symptoms and social functioning. Although psychiatric professionals value the development by users of full insight, this often has a negative impact on self-esteem. This may be avoided by helping users to gain a sense of mastery over their illness, an aim that should be given high priority by professionals.

Encouraging creative activities by users, such as art, theatre performances and poetry, and bringing these into the public arena, is a way of improving the attitudes of the public and enabling users to feel valued. The increasing power of users through the creation of national organisations and a flattening of the hierarchy between professionals and their clients has given users a sense of solidarity and effectiveness in combating institutionalised stigma. However, it is also necessary for the public to make positive efforts to integrate users socially. In view of their moral basis, it is incumbent on religious organisations to participate in this. Befriending schemes run by voluntary groups and adult education classes can also contribute to the increased social inclusion of users.

Part II

Overcoming obstacles to employment

Why work helps

9.1 Why bother about work?

Why should we focus on employment for people with mental illness? One of the most important reasons is that, in the eyes of many people with mental illness, and their friends, family members and treating professionals, work is a fundamental measure of recovery. Among the key concepts of the modern recovery movement is the expectation that the person with mental illness will have a meaningful social role and set of life activities and that he or she will be able to take charge of his or her life and illness. The opportunity to return to a productive role has real meaning for people recovering from psychosis – they become more fully integrated into the life of their community, their relations with friends and family become normalised and the person's self-image is repaired.

Work

They say idleness is the devil's workshop, and that's really true. Having nothing to do during the day except read, and do whatever you want, was not healthy for me. I needed a job or a class. At work I see the same people every day, so I can build a relationship. I didn't really have that before, and being a loner, people pick up on it; they think you're an oddball, and it prevents them making a connection with you. They say, 'We don't know you, maybe you're a dangerous person', or something like that. It has a lot of negativity attached to it, to be alone.

Freud (1930) saw the ability to love and to work as central issues in the lives of men and women. Theodore Roosevelt (1903) believed 'Far and away the best prize that life offers is the chance to work hard at work worth doing.' Primo Levi, who survived Auschwitz and wrote movingly about the experience, believed that humans, even in extreme circumstances, have a need to perform 'work done well' (Roth, 1997). Work is a natural, expected activity for adults in any society, part of being a complete person and a source of identity. Most people with mental illness in Western society want to be working. A job, especially a rewarding one, brings benefits – increased income, expanded social contacts and a sense of meaning in life. Looked at another way, unemployment, for both mentally healthy people and mentally ill people, brings heightened risks of alienation, apathy, substance abuse, physical ill-health and isolation (Bond, 2004a; Warr, 1987). An additional reason to consider work rehabilitation as important is that treatment costs are lower for people with mental illness who are working. Indeed, when a treatment system begins to focus on work as an important outcome and on vocational rehabilitation as a necessary treatment modality, the entire system of care can undergo a transformation into one that is oriented more towards the individual's strengths and future potential (Bond, 2004b).

Work

I really enjoy my job. It isn't really glamorous, but I work at the university and I see a lot of people. I enjoy working with the college students and hanging out with them. I enjoy the whole atmosphere, all the stuff that is going on. I go to a lot of the entertainment and the talks. I'm involved in a lot of the organisations, the political stuff. I just enjoy all the functions of the university and I just feel part of it, even though I don't make a lot of money.

What holds us back from focusing on work as a goal for people with mental illness? Throughout much of the twentieth century, there was a general lack of interest within psychiatry in vocational rehabilitation, in large part because little work was available for people with psychosis. In recent decades, rates of employment for people with psychosis enrolled in standard treatment services in the USA and Britain have rarely exceeded 15% (Bailey et al., 1998; Chandler et al., 1997; Office of National Statistics, 1995). There have been three big obstacles to employment for people with mental illness: high rates of general unemployment, except for some relatively circumscribed periods of labour shortage; the stigma of mental illness, which leads to discrimination against hiring people with mental illness; and, in the post-war decades, disincentives to employment created by the disability pension systems. Consequently, many mental health professionals have discounted the possibility that people with serious mental illness will be able to work, have underestimated the potential value of vocational services (Bond, 2001), and have minimised the importance of work in the lives of their clients. A study in Arkansas revealed that people with schizophrenia rate employment as a much higher priority among their life goals than their mental health care providers rate it as a priority for them (Fischer *et al.*, 2002). Professionals argue variously that their clients are too disabled, not ready for work, afraid of working or too likely to relapse under the stress of working. As we shall see, however, research on modern vocational methods shows these fears to be often unfounded and that high rates of employment for people with mental illness can be achieved, even when competition for jobs is high and when the clients are significantly disabled.

Work

After working full-time this summer there's not enough for me to do. I'm still looking for another situation – something where I can work a 40-hour week. Because that keeps you from dropping back into the stagnant loop where there's just not much happening.

People with mental illness may hold back from working, or their family members may discourage it. One of their most significant concerns – loss of disability benefits – will be examined in the next chapter. The stereotype of mental illness may breed the assumption, accepted even by those afflicted with illness, that they should not work. Consequently, some people with mental illness are afraid of failure or of having to work in close contact with others. For this reason, ongoing support and counselling have to be components of work rehabilitation services.

Role responsibility as a motivation to recovery

They were going to put Bob in a nursing home because his MS was pretty severe. I said, 'Don't do that. I'll take a nursing course and I'll come out and take care of him.' So I did. I spent six months getting my CNA license and I came out here to Colorado. Knowing that I was responsible for Bob and my other patient was kind of like having children. You know, if you have children a lot of times you would have a nervous breakdown, but you don't have it because you've got these kids to take care of. So it was the same for me. There were times when I thought, 'Boy I'm really losing it. I have to go to the hospital.' But I had these two people to take care of so I just stopped the progression, and sometimes I took extra medicine.

9.2 Macro-statistical evidence for benefits of work on the course of schizophrenia

There is good evidence that being productively employed helps people to recover from schizophrenia and other psychotic disorders, but much of this evidence is macro-statistical in scale. That is, we can see the benefits by looking at how people with psychotic illness are affected by large-scale social and economic changes. Let us examine some of this evidence.

Hospital admissions for schizophrenia and other psychotic illnesses increase regularly during economic slumps. This was demonstrated by a US statistician, Harvey Brenner, in his groundbreaking book *Mental Illness and the Economy* (Brenner, 1973). Brenner analysed admissions to New York state mental hospitals, both public and private, from the mid 1800s to the late 1960s, looking for correlations with unemployment rates and other economic indicators. He found that admission rates regularly increased during economic downturns. The relationship was especially clear for patients suffering from functional psychotic illnesses, such as schizophrenia and manic-depressive illness, and held true for both first admissions and later admissions. The effect of economic change was more or less immediate; the admission rate went up as soon as the unemployment rate increased, but the relationship was even stronger one year after the increase. The relationship was specific for the functional psychoses and did not hold true for older patients with dementia. Brenner's work has held up under close scrutiny and has been confirmed by later researchers (Marshall and Funch, 1979; Dear *et al.*, 1979; Parker, 1979; Ahr *et al.*, 1981).

Brenner offered three possible explanations for the association between increased unemployment and increasing admissions of people with psychosis. First, family members' tolerance for a mentally ill relative might decrease as families encounter greater economic stress. The data do not support this hypothesis, because the most dependent – the young and the elderly – are more likely to be hospitalised in the boom and not in the recession. A second possibility is that financial hardship drives people with mental illness to seek the shelter of hospital as if it were an almshouse. Again, this explanation is not supported by the facts. Higher-social-class patients show the same increase in admission rates during the slump as do poorer patients, and admissions to expensive private hospitals also increase during recessions, bringing an increased economic burden, not relief. We are left with one likely explanation – unemployment and economic stress lead to an increase in symptoms of psychosis. How might this work? People with schizophrenia and related psychoses, or those who are susceptible to these disorders, are more likely to be functioning marginally on the job and to be laid off when the economy takes a downturn; the stress of job loss (or of increased contact with stress-inducing relatives) could trigger the development of psychotic symptoms. The fact that it is principally working-age men and women who show increased hospital admissions during the economic downturn makes this more likely.

Outcome from schizophrenia worsens during major economic downturns. Warner (2004) conducted a meta-analysis of the outcome studies of schizophrenia carried out in the developed world during the twentieth century. The meta-analytic approach combines all the subjects from selected, previously conducted research studies into one sample in order to look at the averaged data for the large group of subjects. This meta-analysis encompassed 114 studies conducted between 1912 and 2000 and reporting outcomes for patients admitted between 1898 and 1993 who were diagnosed with schizophrenia or schizophreniform disorder. The total number of subjects for whom usable data were available was over 14 500. The study samples were comprised of subjects selected at the point of admission to hospital or outpatient treatment. Samples included adolescent and adult patients and patients who were early in the illness and those who were long-term sufferers. The length of follow-up varied from study to study, from one year at the shortest to 40 years or until death at the longest. The analysis coded whether the subject was in or out of hospital at follow-up, whether the subject had achieved 'social recovery' (economic and residential independence and low social disruption) and whether the subject had achieved a 'complete recovery' (loss of psychotic symptoms and return to the pre-illness level of functioning). The data were analysed in 15- or 20-year consecutive time periods corresponding to major economic and social changes, one of which was the Great Depression of the 1920s and 1930s.

The analysis showed that there was a good rate of recovery from schizophrenia throughout the twentieth century – around 20% complete recovery and 40% social recovery – but that these recovery rates were much reduced during the Great Depression to around 10% complete recovery and 30% social recovery. Throughout the twentieth century, there was a statistical association between the rate of employment and recovery from schizophrenia. In both the USA and the UK, the two countries in which the majority of the studies were conducted, the rate of recovery was correlated inversely and significantly correlated with the unemployment rate during the period in which the patients were admitted (see Figure 9.1).

The outcome results for Britain are particularly striking. During the decades immediately after the Second World War, Britain was suffering from an acute labour shortage. *The Times* of London called for the immigration of half a million foreign workers and the cabinet of the government discussed banning the football pools (a popular national gambling enterprise) to force the redeployment of the women who processed the coupons into the labour-starved textile industry. At this point in history, Britain launched a social psychiatry revolution that transformed the hospital wards into more stimulating and humanising

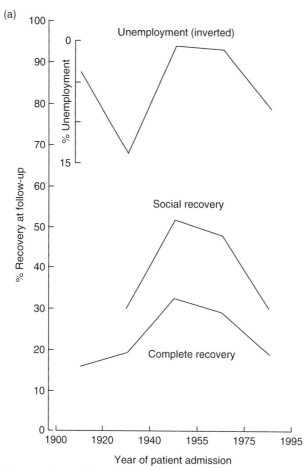

Figure 9.1   Outcome from schizophrenia in (a) the UK and (b) the USA as reflected in 67 studies (33 in the UK and 34 in the USA) of patients admitted between 1901 and 1995, and average unemployment (inverted) for five time periods in the twentieth century. From Warner (2004).

environments, developed work-training schemes and began to move long-hospitalised patients into the community. This revolution in the care of mentally ill people was evident only in northern European countries with full employment – Britain, Norway, Switzerland and the Netherlands – and did not happen to anything like the same extent in the USA, where unemployment was running high. The outcome from schizophrenia in Britain improved to greater heights at this time than has been seen anywhere in the modern developed world, before or since – over 30% full recovery and over 50% social recovery at long-term

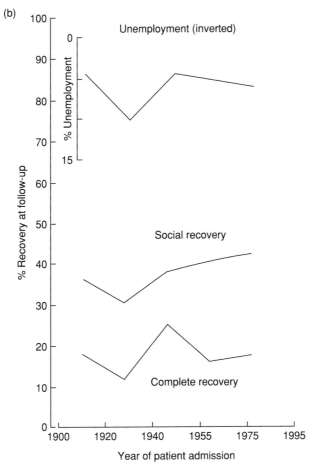

Figure 9.1   (*cont.*)

follow-up. When unemployment rates rose severely in the last two decades of the twentieth century in Britain, however, recovery rates in schizophrenia declined substantially, to less than 20% full recovery and 30% social recovery. Throughout this period, vocational services for people with mental illness were limited. Many people with psychosis were homeless, and the proportion of jail inmates who were suffering from psychosis increased substantially (Warner, 2004).

Interestingly, funding for mental health services does not usually decrease when the economy is doing poorly. In fact, the reverse – increased spending on psychiatric services – is more common. This was the case in Britain during the high unemployment years at the end of the twentieth century (Warner, 2004). So, it is likely that the labour market has a direct effect on services for people with psychosis. Rehabilitative efforts for people with serious mental illness become more assertive during times of labour shortage and less oriented towards helping them find work when unemployment is running high. Not surprisingly, the overall outcome from schizophrenia appears to follow these trends in service provision.

Outcome from schizophrenia is better in the developing world. As we pointed out in Chapter 2, studies conducted by the WHO in several developed and developing countries have demonstrated the unexpected finding that outcome from psychosis is consistently better in the developing world, particularly in rural settings, compared with in the developed West. We cannot be sure why this is case. One explanation offered in Chapter 2 is that the family's emotional responses to people with psychosis are different in developed and developing countries. Another explanation is that people recovering from psychosis in a village subsistence agricultural economy are likely to be readily accepted back into a productive role, something that does not happen in wage-labour settings until the person has regained his or her full functioning capacity or something close to it.

Outcome in psychosis is better for people from the higher social classes in the developed world, but for those from the lower social classes in the developing world. The social classes that come off worst in the competition for jobs in the developed world are the poorest. Unemployment of black people in the USA, for example, is regularly twice that of white people, in good times or bad. Unemployment is tougher on unskilled people, as they may fall off the job ladder, while people in higher occupational classes can take jobs at a lower level of skill and responsibility. It is also true that recovery from psychosis is worst in the lower socio-economic groups in the developed countries. This has been demonstrated many times, beginning with studies in Britain (Cooper, 1961) and the USA (Hollingshead and Redlich, 1958) in the 1950s and continuing to more recent times (Myers and Bean, 1968; Astrachan *et al.*, 1974; World Health Organization, 1979). There are a number of possible explanations for this social-class gradient in outcome from psychosis, including the effects of economic hardship, different levels of acceptance for people with mental illness in the family and the community, and labour-market stress.

Economic hardship, however, cannot explain the curious finding that in the developing world, poorly educated farmers have the better outcome from schizophrenia, and upper-class and upper-caste citizens do worse (World Health Organization, 1979). It could well be that better family and community tolerance (as we suggested in Chapter 2) and reduced labour-market stresses work to the advantage of lower-class people with psychosis in the developing world. Those employed in subsistence farming, with the easiest road back to productive work, are from the lowest classes. It is the members of the urban upper class who are more likely to be exposed to high rates of unemployment in the developing world wage-labour force.

This macro-statistical evidence suggests that the opportunity for productive employment may be a factor leading to improved outcome in psychosis. Let us see whether there is evidence at the individual level.

9.3   Evidence of benefits of work at the individual level

Until the 1990s, because of professional pessimism about the possibility of finding work for clients, little research was conducted on the impact of work on individuals with mental illness. Vocational services and employment outcomes were so poor through the latter part of the twentieth century that the results discouraged further research. Recent advances in the field have stimulated a resurgence of interest, however, and the subsequent research has addressed two major questions: Are rehabilitation programmes effective in getting people with mental illness back to work? And do people with serious mental illness do better and have a milder course of illness if they are employed? In Chapter 11 we will review the evidence for the effectiveness of modern vocational programmes in keeping people employed. Here, we will address whether people with mental illness who are employed do better.

Work and self-esteem

My horizons have broadened. I'm gaining confidence daily, some financial security – not great but I'm earning something. I took my first paycheque – it was my first in seven years – and I framed it. I photocopied it because I had to cash it, but I put the copy in a frame in my home. Then I wrote a personal cheque and put it in a smaller frame. I feel plugged in to society because I'm working. I'm gaining friendships so my isolation is limited. I may self-isolate for a weekend but that's more or less like downtime to recoup.

Before the recent era of randomised controlled research of vocational services, several studies demonstrated that people with psychotic illness who were working fared better than those who were not working. It was unclear, however, whether employment led to clinical improvement or whether higher functioning had made employment possible for some people (Brown *et al.*, 1958; Freeman and Simmons, 1963; Anthony *et al.*, 1972). As vocational programmes became more effective and controlled studies were conducted, however, not only work-related improvements but also clinical and social benefits were noted. People involved in vocational rehabilitation were, for example, more likely to engage in activities with friends, to perform well in social and family roles, to own a driver's licence, to take their antipsychotic medication regularly and to drink less alcohol. Since the early 1990s, a series of studies have identified more and more benefits for people with mental illness who are working. These studies have demonstrated that participation in an effective vocational programme or having paid employment reduces psychiatric hospital admissions (Drake *et al.*, 1996; Bell *et al.*, 1996; Warner *et al.*, 1999; Brekke *et al.*, 1999) and health-care costs (Bond *et al.*, 1995; Warner *et al.*, 1999) and results in a decrease in both positive and negative symptoms of psychosis (Anthony *et al.*, 1995; Bell *et al.*, 1996; McFarlane *et al.*, 2000; Bond, 2001). Similarly, successful work programmes lead to an increase in the participant's quality of life (Mueser *et al.*, 1997a; Holzner *et al.*, 1998; Warner *et al.*, 1999; Bryson *et al.*, 2002; Mueser *et al.*, 2004), to improvements in self-esteem (Brekke *et al.*, 1993; Mueser *et al.*, 1997a; Kates *et al.*, 1997; Bond *et al.*, 2001; Casper and Fishbein, 2002), to an increase in the client's level of functioning (Mueser *et al.*, 1997a; Brekke *et al.*, 1999; Mueser *et al.*, 2004) and to an expansion of the client's social network (Angell and Test, 2002).

It is important to note that the common concern of clinicians – that patients with serious mental illness will become more disturbed under the stress of working – has not proven true. Hospital admissions, symptoms and suicide attempts do not increase when patients are involved in effective work rehabilitation schemes (Bond *et al.*, 2001).

We can look at some of this research in more detail. One study that shows that work leads to symptom reduction in schizophrenia was conducted in the mid 1990s by Morris Bell and his associates. These researchers placed 150 people with schizophrenia in six-month work placements in a Veterans Administration medical centre in Connecticut and assigned them randomly to either being unpaid or being paid US $3.40 an hour. As expected, the people who were paid worked more hours. In addition, those who were paid showed more improvement in their symptoms, particularly emotional discomfort and positive symptoms, such as hallucinations and delusions, and were less likely to be readmitted to hospital. The more the patients worked, the more their symptoms were reduced (Bell *et al.*, 1996). The wage programme was discontinued after six months, but the condition of the patients was followed up again six months later. Three-quarters of the patients who had worked for pay continued to work as volunteers or paid. Those who had been in paid employment during the first six months of the programme were still less disturbed by symptoms of psychosis and emotional discomfort at 12-months' follow-up (Bell and Lysaker, 1997).

Another study that shows a progressively improving course of illness for people with serious mental illness who gain employment was conducted in Boulder,

Colorado. Thirty-eight people with psychotic disorders who were attending the Chinook Clubhouse, a psychosocial clubhouse that placed members in supported employment, were matched with an equal number of people with similar disorders who lived too far away to be able to attend the clubhouse but who were in the same community psychiatry treatment service. After two years, the clubhouse members had achieved higher levels of employment and a better quality of life. Although the costs of treatment of the unemployed people who could not attend the clubhouse increased progressively, the treatment costs for those who achieved employment through the clubhouse decreased substantially, due to a drop in both inpatient and outpatient care, indicating a progressive improvement in disability and course of illness (Warner *et al.*, 1999).

Several other recent US studies have demonstrated clinical benefits for clients who obtain work. Anthony *et al.* (1995) found that for 275 people with mental illness who participated in a rehabilitation programme, those who became employed showed greater improvements in psychiatric symptoms, especially negative symptoms of psychosis. When a New England mental health centre converted its day treatment programme into a supported employment model, the rehospitalisation rate of the 112 clients with serious mental illness who were affected by the change was halved in the year following the transition (Drake *et al.*, 1996). Mueser and associates (1997a) found that in a group of nearly 150 unemployed patients who enrolled in a rehabilitation programme, those who were working at 18-months' follow-up had less severe symptoms of thought disorder and affective disturbance, higher functioning, greater satisfaction with aspects of their lives, and better self-esteem than unemployed patients. Bond and colleagues (2001) conducted a study of nearly 150 people with severe mental illness to see whether employment led to improvements in other areas. They concluded that those who engaged in competitive work showed greater improvement in symptoms, in leisure activities, in their finances and in self-esteem than those who were not working.

Research shows increasing support for the suggestion that the availability of employment improves outcome in psychosis, and it is likely that the evidence for this thesis would be more impressive if the available research studies were not so short in duration. Most of the studies are conducted over 6–12 months, and few are continued for longer than 18 months. Bond and colleagues (2001) argue that longer periods of study are needed to uncover the clinical benefits of sustained work – in other words, the effects of employment are cumulative and become stronger the longer a person is working. It is, in fact, usually the longer-term studies, i.e. those that run for 18 months or longer, that have demonstrated clinical benefits for the participants (Mueser *et al.*, 1997a; McFarlane *et al.*, 2000; Bond *et al.*, 2001). Studies of people with schizophrenia enrolled in rehabilitation programmes often show that clinical outcomes improve progressively over time (Brekke *et al.*, 1999; Warner *et al.*, 1999; Mueser *et al.*, 2004). Research can be expensive, and long-term studies even more so. Consequently, most research is of short duration, which means that we do not know as much as we should about the impact of work, social factors or treatment interventions on long-term disorders. Psychiatrists Greden and Tandon (1995, p. 197), in evaluating this problem, conclude that 'our knowledge gaps about long-term . . . treatment may be the most important issue faced by psychiatry today'.

We should also note that all of the work-related research has been conducted on people who have been ill for substantial periods of time – people for whom the symptoms and course of illness have long been established – and not on people who are in the early stages of psychosis and for whom a rapid return to a productive role might be more likely to make a difference to the long-term course of the disorder. If we are to understand the full impact that work can have on the symptoms and course of psychotic illness, we may have to put into place programmes that help provide employment for people with serious disorders from the earliest stages of their illnesses and research programmes that follow their condition over extended periods of time.

Comparative research results, although essential, do not tell us the whole story. Changes can occur in the culture of a treatment service that affect clients, families and staff alike, as more of those who suffer from a psychosis become employed. One of us (RW) has worked in the same system of care in Boulder county, Colorado, for nearly 30 years. During that time, he has seen improvements in the local economy, in the services, in the employment status of the clients, and in the attitudes of staff and service users. During the lean years and the oil crisis of the Carter administration in the late 1970s, treatment and rehabilitation services were developed poorly and less than 15% of people with a psychosis were employed. An early 1980s survey of Boulder clients with psychosis revealed that the biggest problem they reported was boredom and their greatest need was employment (Fromkin, 1985). Even in the early 1990s, more than half of these clients reported that they had nothing to do each day other than come to the treatment agency for an hour or less (Warner *et al.*, 1994). Beyond that, the only activities to fill the hours between rising and going to bed were hanging out with friends and smoking marijuana, panhandling for spare change or sitting alone in an empty apartment watching TV. One of the clinicians' greatest concerns was the epidemic of drug abuse among their clients with mental illness. By 2000, the last year of the Clinton administration and the high-tech bubble, however, change was evident. There was full employment in Boulder county. Employers were much more keen to hire people with mental illness and, thanks to a variety of vocational services and the activities of a psychosocial clubhouse, half of the adult clients with a psychosis were employed. The common client culture was no longer one of isolation, idleness and drug use but one of work, study or related activities and social engagement. The staff of the agency, in consequence, had become more focused on ways to increase the independence and quality of life of their clients with mental illness.

9.4   Conclusions

Work is a fundamentally important part of everyone's life, no less the lives of people with mental illness. As such, it is seen by many, including people with mental illness, their carers and their treatment providers, as an essential measure of recovery. A focus on work can reorient an entire treatment system towards the future potential of its clients and can reinforce the clients' optimism about recovery.

Many factors, however, hold us back from focusing on work rehabilitation. High rates of general unemployment and discrimination against employing people with mental illness, coupled with the disincentives to employment created by the disability pension schemes, have led to low rates of employment for people with mental illness. This has caused mental health professionals and others to become pessimistic about reemployment. Until recently, vocational services have been adapted poorly to the needs of people with mental illness, but, as we shall see in Chapter 11, this no longer has to be the case.

It is worth focusing on work, as there is a good deal of evidence that working helps people to recover from mental illness. Much of the evidence is macro-social in nature – for example, business cycles appear to have an effect on hospital admission rates for psychosis and on outcome from schizophrenia. At the individual level, moreover, recent research shows that working can lead to less frequent admission to hospital, lower symptoms of psychosis, lower treatment costs, improved quality of life, improved social functioning and enlarged social networks. It is becoming clear, however, that if we are to see the full benefits of work and vocational programmes, then we need to intervene early in the illness and to follow people for longer periods of time after they become employed.

These are the potential rewards. In the next chapter, we will look at how we might overcome some of the obstacles to employment that stand in the way of people with mental illness.

Economic obstacles to employment

10.1 Disincentives to employment in entitlement programmes

When a person suffers from serious mental illness, his or her decisions, including economic decisions, are sometimes dismissed as irrational. A decision not to work may be seen as evidence of lack of drive or depressive feelings of inadequacy. Failure to hold a job for long may be thought of as due to functional deficits from the illness. Refusal to consider a low-paid job may be considered a result of negativism, grandiose aspirations or lack of insight into one's true functional ability. Squandering one's disability income long before the end of the month might be regarded as an example of poor judgement secondary to psychosis. Liebow's (1967) study of the inner-city poor, however, illustrates that these problems are not specific to people with mental illness but are common responses to poverty and to the work opportunities available to poor people.

In the years before the Second World War, psychiatrists were misled into identifying certain behaviours of hospitalised mentally ill people, such as mannerisms, posturing, pacing and mutism, as typical features of schizophrenia. These behaviours were shown later to be largely a result of institutional confinement. We can learn from this mistake. Today, a better understanding of the economic condition of people with mental illness in the community may help us clarify the extent to which symptoms of psychiatric patients are an integral part of the illness or are determined environmentally. We need to know, for example, to what degree the low self-esteem, withdrawal, apathy and anxiety we see in people with schizophrenia are negative symptoms of the illness or are the long-recognised consequences of long-term unemployment (Eisenberg and Lazarsfeld, 1938).

Perhaps because people with mental illness tend to be seen as inherently irrational, there have been few attempts to examine their economic behaviour, incentives, choices and economic realities. Some publications have addressed the economic impact of schizophrenia on society (Gunderson and Mosher,

1975; McGuire, 1991; Moscarelli *et al.*, 1996) and on the patient's family (Hart, 1982; McGuire, 1991), and others have addressed the economic decision-making of physically disabled people (Berkowitz and Hill, 1986), but few have examined the economic decision-making of people with mental illness (Bell *et al.*, 1993; Turton, 2001; Drew *et al.*, 2001). In fact, when the available economic choices are made clear, the financial decisions of people with mental illness can be readily understood. As anyone might, people with mental illness ask themselves: What are my income options? How much effort is required to generate how much income?

In order to evaluate the extent to which economic factors influence the life choices of people with mental illness, one of us (RW), along with economic development specialist Paul Polak, interviewed 50 people with mental illness living in Boulder, Colorado, in 1992 (Polak and Warner, 1996). Using a standard-ised interview format, we asked subjects about their cash income from earnings, disability pension, gifts, loans, illegal activities and other sources and for details of their non-cash income from rent subsidies and donated items such as food, clothes, medication and services. We asked the subjects about their economic decision-making. Why were some sources of cash or non-cash income rejected? What were the disincentives and incentives for working? How much did the subject need to earn in order to make working worthwhile? It became clear that these people faced significant financial disincentives to work. The average total cash and non-cash income of subjects who were employed part-time (US $1028 a month) was only modestly higher than that of unemployed subjects (US $929 a month). The small size of the difference was due largely to the fact that most subjects lost entitlements such as disability pension and rent subsidy when they started to work.

If working doesn't make much economic sense, then this could help explain why in recent decades in the USA and Britain, only about 15% of people with serious mental illness have been employed (Anthony *et al.*, 1988; Consumer Health Sciences, 1997; Office of National Statistics, 1995; Turton, 2001). Employ-ment rates for people with mental illness may be influenced by the availability of employment, the provision of vocational rehabilitation services and work disincentives in the disability pension system. In this chapter, we will be looking primarily at the last of these factors.

One further factor – the limitations imposed by the illness itself – can be quantified and set aside. It is clear that 50–60% of people with schizophrenia and other forms of psychosis can work in the competitive workforce. In northern Italy, for example, a substantial proportion of people with psychosis are employed. In Bologna and Verona in the mid 1990s, 50% or more of people with schizophrenia were working, 20–25% of them full-time (Warner *et al.*, 1998). Later in this chapter, we will take a look at the way in which the Italian disability benefit system imposes fewer work disincentives. In the USA, supported-employment research programmes for people with serious mental illness routinely achieve employment rates of 50–60%. In the non-research setting of Boulder, Colorado, during the economic boom of 2000, with strong vocational programmes in place, over half of all the public mental health centre's clients with psychosis were in paid employment. It is clear that it is not psychosis per se that imposes the grievously high rates of idleness, but the economic system within which we function.

Economic disincentives to work

I'm upset that if I make much money, I'll lose all my benefits. If I get a good job, I'll lose my health insurance, and if I lose my Medicaid, my medicines will cost me $2000 a month. If you get a good job and become productive and successful for a while and then become mentally ill again and lose your job, you have absolutely no safety net. You know it's very scary to get off all the programmes when you don't know what's going to happen, especially with the economy and stuff. It really scares me to try becoming totally self-sufficient. I think the system is very unfair and flawed.

Let us look more closely at the obstacles imposed by the disability benefits system. In the USA, there are two major governmental disability support programmes – supplemental security income (SSI) and social security disability income (SSDI). The rules governing each are complex, but they can be simplified as follows. Under both programmes, support payments decline when a disabled person accepts employment. Recipients of SSI lose 50 cents of benefits for each dollar earned when earnings exceed US$65–85 a month. Those receiving a rent subsidy encounter further losses. Economists refer to this loss of income with increasing earned income as an 'implicit tax'. SSDI recipients lose nothing until they earn over US$700 a month, and then they lose it all.

The way the implicit tax works can be illustrated by the hypothetical case of two disabled people, one on SSI and another on SSDI, each receiving US$512 monthly in disability income and US$400 in rent subsidy. If each were to take a job working 15 hours a week at US$6 an hour, then the SSI recipient would make an overall gain of US$156/month, or US$2.59 for each hour worked (implicit tax = 57%); the SSDI recipient would gain US$252/month, or US$4.20 for each work hour (implicit tax = 30%). The SSDI recipient benefits more from each hour worked, until the monthly income exceeds US$700, at which point he or she loses all the disability benefits and drops below the income of the SSI recipient, until he or she was working many more hours a week. Polak and Warner (1996) interviewed a second sample of people with psychosis in 1994 – this time, 100 randomly selected subjects – about their work status, income and wage requirements. In this study, the implicit tax associated with accepting part-time employment averaged 64% – higher than in the examples cited here because of loss of additional benefits such as food stamps and free medicines. Thus, a person working part-time for minimum wage (US$4.25 an hour at that time) would actually have kept, in real terms, US$1.57 an hour. To understand why so few people with psychosis are working, try hiring a babysitter for US$1.57 (at the time of writing, less than £1) an hour; even in 1994 you wouldn't have found many takers.

Here is an illustration of how a real person with schizophrenia in Boulder dealt with these economic issues:

Jennifer, a 28-year-old single woman with schizo-affective disorder, was receiving the SSI pension of US$409 a month. She took a 25-hour-a-week job as a teacher's aide for developmentally disabled children, earning US$6.63 an hour. In so doing, her SSI dropped by US$315 a month, she lost US$17 a month in food stamps and her rent subsidy went down by US$143. Now that she was working, she could no longer stop at her parents' house and eat lunch every day, and she was often too tired to go there to eat at night. As a result, the cost of her food and meals went up by US$110 a month. Overall, she found herself ahead by no more than US$73 a month. The decision to continue in the job became based, therefore, not on economic gains, which were insignificant, but on the opposing factors of stress and self-esteem. Initially, because the disabled pupil to whom she was assigned was so difficult, she decided she would quit. When she was given an easier child to work with, however, Jennifer resolved to continue in the job. Without an analysis of her economic situation, her ambivalence about working would not have appeared as rational as, in fact, it was, and might have been blamed on schizophrenic apathy, deficits in functioning or just plain laziness.

In our study of 100 people with psychosis, the situation seemed to be better for full-time workers. Full-time workers met an implicit tax of only 23% and, after deducting the implicit tax, kept an average of US$5 an hour of their earnings. Many people with mental illness, however, are incapable of moving straight into full-time work.

In response to these disincentives, most mentally disabled people identify a minimum earnings level that makes work an economically sensible choice – what economists term their 'reservation wage'. More than three-quarters of the clients we surveyed in Boulder in 1992 ruled out the option of taking a job at the official minimum wage (at that time US$4.25 an hour), but over 60% were willing to work for US$5 an hour; 80% would have worked for US$6 an hour (Polak and Warner, 1996). We concluded that in order to employ significant numbers of people with mental illness in Boulder, we would need to find or create jobs that paid above the minimum wage, or the government would need to change the disincentives in the benefits system. In this chapter and those that follow, we will be looking at how each of these goals might be achieved.

10.2 National variations in disability benefits systems

In Britain, disincentives to work are worse than in the USA. British disabled people run the risk of losing all their incapacity benefit (over £75 a week) if they earn more than £78 a week. This earnings disregard is permitted for only six months, with some possibility of extension. People receiving a different disability benefit are allowed to earn no more than £20 a week before losing their income support. Most disabled people, moreover, receive other care allowances and means-tested benefits, such as housing benefit, which, for someone with dependants, can exceed £200 a week. These added benefits are reduced as soon as the disabled person earns more than £20 a week. Since a full benefits package, including disability pension, housing subsidy and free prescriptions, is worth about £14 000 a year, tax-free, and a full-time minimum-wage job yields only £10 000 a year of taxable income, there is little incentive for psychiatrically disabled people to work part-time or full-time (Turton, 2001; Grove, 2004).

Various attempts have been made to alleviate these disincentives in the UK, but with little success. One measure allows the disabled person to return automatically to the same level of benefits if his or her job ends within a year. Another measure, the Working Tax Credit, tops up incomes for working people who earn less than £14 600 a year and provides free prescriptions. Despite these measures, nearly a million Britons with psychiatric impairments, at least half of whom would prefer to be in paid work, are receiving incapacity benefits. Less than 5% of those who have been receiving incapacity benefit for two years return to the labour market (Grove, 2004).

In Italy, work disincentives are generally less severe than in the USA or Britain because (i) fewer people with mental illness qualify for a disability pension and (ii) Italian disabled people often manage to retain their disability benefits while working. The disability benefit of €500 a month (at the time of writing, £340 or $650) is a little higher than in the USA and substantially lower than in Britain, but this is not the critical issue – to receive the financial benefit, the person must be over '79% disabled'. A system of this sort is possible only because 80–90% of Italians with psychosis are living with, and being supported by, their families. This absence of formal income support for many people with mental illness increases the incentive to make use of the work opportunities that are often quite comprehensive for people with mental illness in Italy, especially in the north of the country. These opportunities are made available through the

disability system (Law 68), through direct employment, through training programmes (*borse lavoro*) and through special worker cooperatives linked to the
psychiatric services, which will be described in Chapter 12 (Fioritti, 2004).
The combination of reduced disincentives and increased opportunities leads
to the substantially higher rates of employment for Italians with mental illness
already cited above.

Beyond these formal system features, however, many Italian people with
mental illness who receive disability benefits continue to work in the black-
market labour force. In Italian seaside resorts, for example, many psychiatrically
disabled people find temporary jobs along the beaches. In rural areas, they
may work on family farms. Black-market employment is so common and
well-recognised that European psychiatric researchers code it as 'competitive
employment' as long as it does not involve drug-dealing.

Work disincentives are less severe in Greece for a different reason – the
disability pension is so low that working is a better option. The Greek disability
pension is less than US$150 a month, and a minimum-wage job brings in four
times as much.

Economic disincentives to work

I work under the table at one of my jobs. I can't report it to social security, but if
I want to have a car I have to have money for the insurance, the upkeep, eventually
a car. So I work two jobs. One of them the government doesn't know about and
hopefully won't find out about.

10.3 What should be changed? Proposals for system reform

How can research help?

'Everybody talks about the weather but nobody does anything about it.' This
aphorism, attributed to Mark Twain, could apply equally well to the disability
benefits system. If we are to do something about the problem of disincentives, we
will need some research guidance about what changes in social policy will
increase employment for people with mental illness.

Econometric labour-supply models (Moffit, 1990) can be used to forecast the
effects of changes in incapacity benefits policy on people with disability. This type
of computer modelling requires the collection of data on work and income from a
sample that is large enough to provide examples of a substantial number of
people in different categories of work/income budget constraints. Averett *et al.*

(1999) gathered economic information from over 200 randomly selected people with psychotic disorders in treatment with the mental health centre in Boulder, Colorado. We looked at what would happen if the regulations governing the US disability pension programme, SSI, were modified. (SSI is the programme in which recipients lose 50 cents of pension for each dollar earned when earnings exceed US$65–85 a month.) The model revealed something fairly obvious: that unearned income was a significant disincentive to working or to increasing one's hours of work. It also demonstrated that providing a wage subsidy was one of the most effective ways to boost working hours. In our computer model, offering a wage subsidy of US$2 (about £1.05) an hour led to an increase of more than 5% in weekly hours of work. In addition, increasing the earnings disregard – the amount of money that a starting worker can earn before losing money from the SSI cheque – was beneficial. Doubling the earnings disregard under SSI (US$65 a month) improved work hours by 3%; increasing it to US$1000 a month boosted working hours by 11%. By contrast, changing SSI regulations to reduce the rate of loss of income support as people increased their hours of work (currently 50 cents in the dollar) – that is, reducing the implicit tax on earned income – was surprisingly ineffective in boosting hours of work.

These findings suggest two possible social policy innovations: (i) increasing the amount of earned income that would be allowed before the disability pension is reduced and (ii) providing a wage subsidy.

Raising the earnings disregard

Let us take an example. In the USA, the allowable earned income level could be increased from the current US$700 a month under SSDI, and from US$65 under SSI, to $1000 or more a month. In 1999, the earnings disregard under SSDI was, in fact, increased from US$500 to US$700 a month. Although this still did not bring mentally ill and other disabled people up to parity with blind people (for whom the earnings disregard has been over US$1000 a month since 1990), the change, as we shall see, seems to have allowed many disabled people to increase their hours of work and their income.

A study in Boulder County, Colorado, seized the opportunity to see what happens to the employment and income of people with serious mental illness when (i) jobs are plentiful, (ii) an effective supported employment programme is in place and (iii) the earnings disregard is increased (Warner et al., 2004). The author and his colleagues surveyed the work and income of two different samples of more than 130 working-age outpatients with psychotic illness, selected randomly at two points in time three years apart, in 1997 and 2000. During this period, the local unemployment rate halved from 3.9% to 2.0% and the earnings disregard under SSDI increased from US$500 to US$700 a month. All the subjects had access to a vigorous supported employment programme operated by a psychosocial clubhouse. What was the result of these improved conditions? The proportion of patients in stable employment increased dramatically from 30% in 1997 to 47% in 2000, indicating that more people with serious mental illness can be employed when the unemployment rate is low and vocational services are good. Patients receiving SSDI benefits showed a significantly greater increase in stable employment (from 35% to 47%) than those receiving SSI (whose employment increased from 23% to 30%). Those receiving SSDI also increased their hours of work, but SSI recipients did not. The results suggest that SSDI, with its high earnings disregard, presented fewer disincentives to employment. Furthermore, the rate of employment and the hours of work of SSDI recipients may well have been boosted by relaxation in the SSDI earnings limitation in 1999.

Although these results are for people receiving US disability pensions, they have broader applicability. The same principle applies to other national disability benefits and to other entitlement programmes. British commentators have called for a revision of the earnings disregard for both income support and housing benefit programmes (Davis and Betteridge, 1997; Disability Income Group, 1997; Simons, 1998; Turton, 2001). Raising the earnings disregard in benefits systems for disabled people could lead more people with serious mental illness to work and improve the course of their illness.

Wage subsidies

We could also consider providing a wage subsidy to the most seriously disabled mentally ill people and thereby raising earned income above the minimum wage (currently US$5.15 an hour in the USA). How could this innovation be funded? One possibility is that government income-support regulations could be modified in order to allow benefit payments to be diverted into wage subsidies. The money would either go directly to the worker or be used to reimburse the employer for the difference between the worker's rate of production and the expected productivity. The US Department of Labor has established a time-study process to measure this productivity differential (Roberts and Ward, 1987).

It is also feasible to divert funding currently used for treatment services into wage subsidies. In the USA, where much of government-funded psychiatric treatment is being converted to a per capita managed-care funding mechanism, it might be profitable to use treatment funds for wage subsidies. Under per capita funding, the treatment agency keeps any savings resulting from programme innovations that reduce costs. For example, a reduction in hospital costs can be directed to community treatment. If increased employment can be shown to improve stability of illness and to reduce treatment costs, then an agency with capitated funding could choose to provide a wage subsidy for its most disabled patients.

Can treatment costs, in fact, be reduced by employing patients? Psychiatric treatment costs were more than twice as high for the unemployed patients in the study conducted in Boulder than for the part-time employed (Polak and Warner, 1996). This could be explained in a number of ways, one being that working patients do better because they are employed and need less treatment. Whatever the explanation, it is clear that the cost of outpatient treatment of unemployed patients is so high in Boulder (around US$3000 a month per patient) that the expense of providing a half-time wage supplement for these clients could be met by a mere 10% reduction in treatment costs. Such a reduction seems possible, if only because the newly employed client would be at work half the week and less available for treatment. Several studies, in fact, have shown that the time spent in day-treatment programmes decreases substantially for patients who transfer to supported employment (Bailey *et al.*, 1998) or other programmes with a vocational component (McFarlane *et al.*, 2000). As we have seen in the previous chapter, moreover, being in a productive role improves the course of a person's illness, which will lead to reduced cost of treatment.

A study conducted in Boulder, Colorado, demonstrated that treatment costs declined progressively over two years in a group of patients who were enrolled as members of a rehabilitation-oriented clubhouse, while these costs remained constant in a matched group of non-clubhouse members (Warner *et al.*, 1999). The treatment-cost reduction for clubhouse members was restricted to those who were placed in work, suggesting that the savings may well have been a result of employment. Similarly, the treatment costs for clients admitted to Thresholds, a psychosocial clubhouse in Chicago, which has a rehabilitation programme with a strong vocational component, were less than three-quarters of the costs for those admitted to a social club with no vocational component (Bond, 1984). In another study, clients with mental illness randomly selected for a programme of accelerated entry into supported employment generated treatment costs that were less than three-quarters of those for similar clients placed in a gradual work entry programme, more than offsetting the increased rehabilitation costs (Bond *et al.*, 1995). Placing mentally ill people in work can save money. However, to realise cost benefits from a wage subsidy, it would be necessary to track costs carefully over time and to ensure that the subsidy was made available only to the most severely disabled patients.

Bolder steps

Such suggestions as raising the earnings disregard and paying a wage subsidy may seem bold, but they are quite limited in scope compared with some of the other options that have been mooted – welfare reform, guaranteed jobs for disabled people, and raising the minimum wage.

Raising the minimum wage for all workers would have a similar impact on people with mental illness as paying people with disabilities a wage subsidy, but it would cost more and would generate more political opposition. Some welfare-reform advocates have argued for a system of time-limited welfare and guaranteed jobs for all (Kaus, 1986; Ellwood, 1988). The welfare-reform legislation passed by the US congress during the Clinton administration in the early 1990s established time-limited welfare and a small increase in the minimum wage, but it did not establish a guaranteed jobs programme. The Italian vocational provisions for people with mental illness, when they have been comprehensively enacted, have achieved these ends more fully – disability income support is provided to only the most disabled people, and the worker cooperatives in the northern Italian cities are equivalent to guaranteed jobs. It would be a grave error, however, to imagine that we could achieve an effective welfare-to-work transition for people with mental illness in Britain and America merely by cutting back on benefits. To do so would merely deepen the level of poverty in which many people with mental illness are living. Guaranteed earned income has to be available as part of any such transition plan.

Less bold steps

Several observers have argued that there are a variety of additional reasons why few people with mental illness are willing to take a chance on working. One is that the intricacies of the benefits system are so convoluted – involving income support, housing allowances, health insurance, tax credits, different earnings disregard levels, and so on – that no reasonable person can understand them without help. Clear and accurate information is not routinely made available to service users, and the users do not always trust the welfare rights officers who advise them about benefits. Many users find that their entitlements do not return to the prior level rapidly enough if they stop working. Voluntary work or enrolling in training may trigger a review of their entitlement to benefits (Turton, 2001; Grove, 2004). These same observers have suggested that the communication difficulties could be reduced by making available personal advisors, some of whom would themselves be people with disabilities, to provide users with individualised information about return-to-work benefits. They recommend that more people with disabilities should be employed in managerial positions in the employment services and suggest that fear of the assessment and review process could be reduced by a redesign of the whole disability assessment process (Turton, 2001; Grove, 2004).

Beyond these considerations, one thing is clear. An understanding of the way in which financial realities influence users' life decisions is essential to helping users with decisions about working. Therapists and case managers who have concerns about a client's process of recovery should have a detailed understanding of the regulations of the benefits system – a level of knowledge that is at least equal to and, we hope, better than their client's own understanding of these fundamentals of modern economic survival.

10.4 Conclusions

People with mental illness living in the developed world face significant financial disincentives to work if they are receiving disability benefits. These disincentives are more severe in Britain and the USA than in Italy, with the result that a much smaller proportion of people with mental illness are employed in the UK and the USA than in Italy. The research suggests that we can reduce the disincentives by raising the amount a disabled person is allowed to earn before benefits are reduced. Providing a wage subsidy to the disabled person is another possible solution. A guaranteed-jobs programme coupled to modifications in the design of the benefits plan could also be successful. Any remedies that are effective in returning seriously mentally people to work could pay for themselves through reductions in treatment costs. No remedies will work, however, unless service users trust that change in employment status will benefit their interests. Personal advisors, who may themselves be users, can help disseminate information about complex benefits-system regulations, and therapists and case managers should understand the regulations well enough to be able to help their clients make good decisions about work and income.

The spectrum of work programmes

11.1 What are the options?

We should be doing more to help people with psychotic illnesses find work and hold on to their jobs. As noted in the previous chapter, 50–60% of people with serious mental illness are capable of employment, but in the USA and Britain no more than 15% of this group is in any kind of paid work. Although 60–70% of Americans with serious mental illness would like to be working, fewer than one-quarter receive any type of vocational assistance (Bond, 2001). Indeed, one US study showed that fewer than 25% of people with psychosis even have a mention of work in their treatment plans (Lehman and Steinwachs, 1998). All this means that about half a million people with schizophrenia in the USA, and about 100 000 people in Britain, are unemployed but potentially productive members of society. One reason for this situation, as we saw in the previous chapter, is the disincentive to work in the disability benefits system. Another is the lack of provision of suitable work opportunities.

In Britain and America, the usual spectrum of employment opportunities for people with mental illness includes the following:

- *Traditional vocational rehabilitation:* clients are referred to an external agency that screens, counsels, trains and places applicants in work and discontinues services when the client is placed.
- *Sheltered workshops:* a widely diffused post-war model developed primarily in northern Europe, regarded by many these days as too institutional and segregated.
- *Supported employment:* this and its close relative, transitional employment, are US models in which jobs are developed for clients in competitive work settings. Training and support for people placed in these jobs are provided on an ongoing basis by staff members known as job coaches.
- *Independent employment:* people with mental illness find jobs in the competitive workforce, with or without the assistance of vocational staff. To these we can add a newer model:

- *Social firms or affirmative businesses:* these are businesses that are created with a dual mission – to create a needed product or service and to employ people with psychiatric disabilities. The model was created in northern Italy in the 1960s in the form of worker cooperatives. It has since diffused into a number of other countries, but it is not yet available widely.

The social enterprise model will be discussed in detail in the next chapter. Here we will review the work programmes that are currently available widely.

Until recently, work rehabilitation for people with serious mental illness didn't seem to work at all well. Two reviews of the research on vocational rehabilitation in psychosis – one by Bond in 1992 and another by Lehman in 1995 – revealed that none of the studies reviewed demonstrated success in improving long-term employment outcomes for people with psychosis until the 1970s (Bond, 1992; Lehman, 1995). Many of the vocational programmes of the 1970s and 1980s were successful in placing people with psychotic illness in sheltered jobs in hospital or elsewhere, or in transitional positions, and in helping them to hold down those jobs, but until the introduction of the supported employment model in the 1990s, not one of these programmes was successful in placing clients in the competitive workforce. Before 1990, the programmes led to increases in paid employment, full-time employment, job starts, duration of employment and earnings, all of which are beneficial, but their meanings to the client are different if the employment is not a permanent job in mainstream society.

Thus, the work programmes of the 1970s and 1980s were able to help the clients adjust to a specific work environment but had no success in getting the person into a 'real job'. The programmes accomplishing these limited ends included work-oriented halfway houses, assertive case-management teams, psychosocial clubhouses and hospital-based programmes – all vocational programmes that were designed specifically for people with mental illness. What most people with mental illness in routine psychiatric treatment were being offered, however, was far less effective – traditional vocational services designed for people with physical rather than psychiatric disabilities. With the introduction of supported employment in the 1990s, mainstream employment became a viable option for people with mental illness. In the best services, this approach began to supplant the ineffective traditional vocational model. It is in the contrast between traditional vocational services – the 'train and place' model – and supported employment – the 'place and train' model – that we see most clearly the breakthrough that has led to success in returning people with mental illness to competitive work.

11.2 Traditional vocational rehabilitation model

In the traditional vocational rehabilitation model, clients with any type of physical or mental disability are referred to an independent agency that screens and assesses applicants, provides them with training and places them in work. Services provided are short-term and success is rated by the number of case 'closures', which occur when clients are placed successfully. There are no on-going services after closure. This pattern of service provision is now regarded as insensitive to the intermittent and ongoing vocational needs of people with serious mental illness. Very few US state vocational rehabilitation agencies, moreover, employ psychiatric rehabilitation staff who can offer specialised services to people with mental illness (Noble *et al.*, 1997). Consumers and family members complain that rehabilitation counsellors spend too much time processing paperwork and too little time providing services after eligibility has been established (Noble *et al.*, 1997). A review of the effectiveness of federal-state vocational rehabilitation programmes by the US General Accounting Office (1993) revealed that few people with mental illness actually receive services from the state vocational agencies, and those that do show no benefit. The analysis found that for clients with mental illness who receive services and are closed as 'successfully rehabilitated', average earnings are less after receiving services than before. The National Alliance for the Mentally Ill argues that the half a billion dollars spent annually in the USA on traditional time-limited services for people with mental illness is a waste of money that could be better spent on more appropriately designed programmes, such as supported employment (Noble, 1998).

11.3 Supported employment and transitional employment

Transitional employment programmes (TEPs) are the precursors of the supported employment approach. TEPs were originally developed in the 1970s by Fountain House, a psychosocial clubhouse in New York City (see Chapter 14), and are still an important element of the clubhouse model. Under this approach, a job coach locates a job in a business or agency in the local community and learns how to do the job. The job coach then trains a person with mental illness to do the job and places him or her in the position for a limited period, usually six months. At the end of that time, a new person is placed in the job. The original incumbent has to find or be placed in a new position. The worker in the TEP position is supported on the job by the job coach and can attend weekly support meetings and evening meals. If the disabled person cannot work at any time, for whatever reason, the job coach will find someone else to work that day or will do the job him-or herself. Consequently, the employer of someone placed through a transitional (or supported) employment programme gets a good deal. He or she knows that the job – often a high-turnover, entry-level position – will be filled permanently and reliably and that the worker training is done by an outside service.

The principle behind transitional employment is that the person with mental illness learns basic job skills in a transitional position that will help him or her to achieve the ultimate goal – a permanent unsupported job in the competitive marketplace. In fact, the research does not support the notion that TEP workers are more likely to secure competitive employment (Lehman, 1995) and, given the extreme sensitivity of people with schizophrenia to the stresses of change, it is hard to believe that transitional employment is ideally suited to this population. In fact, the origins of the TEP idea were not entirely consumer-driven. One of the reasons that programmes such as Fountain House developed the transitional model of employment was that they found it difficult to locate enough jobs and provide ongoing support to all of the clients who wanted work.

More suitable for the person with mental illness, who may not be able to tolerate the stress of job change or to learn new tasks easily, is the supported employment model, developed originally for people with developmental dis-abilities. This model is similar to the TEP approach, except that the job is permanent. As the worker adjusts to the demands of the position, work supports can be gradually decreased and provided to another client placed more recently in work. As a result the number of supported employment positions continues to expand over time. Supported employment offers several advantages. Employ-ment can be designed to meet the needs of each individual client. Job-sharing can be arranged for those who, because of the disincentives in the disability benefits system and the symptom-generating demands of full-time work, prefer to work part-time. Jobs, moreover, can be sought to match the skills and preferences of individual clients, and, since positions are permanent, a career ladder is possible.

Ideally, a supported employment team will include a manager and at least three full-time staff whose time is devoted exclusively to vocational work. When staff are given both clinical and vocational duties, they are likely to be co-opted to provide more and more clinical and case-management services at the expense of the rehabilitation work. The team should be physically located within the mental health centre providing psychiatric services in order to integrate the rehabilitation work with the clinical services. Each staff member has an individual caseload of about 20 consumers, but team members help one another with job leads and other supports. Staff members spend about half of their time out of the office supervising and training clients on site and meeting with employers (Becker and Bond, 2002; Becker and Drake, 2003).

11.4 Individual placement and support

A refinement of the supported employment model is individual placement and support (IPS). Bond (1998; 2004a) has outlined several principles of this approach:

Eligibility is based on consumer choice

No potential clients are excluded because of a poor previous work record, lack of 'work-readiness', frequent hospital admissions or current symptoms. Thus, the IPS approach sidesteps some of the problems associated with traditional vocational services, including the screening out of most people with mental illness and the failure to predict accurately who can work successfully (Noble et al., 1997). People with mental illness have better outcomes in supported employment than other programmes, regardless of such clinical characteristics as diagnosis and previous frequency of hospitalisation. Even clients with disturbed cognitive functioning appear to accommodate successfully to the job with enough assistance from the supported employment programme (McGurk and Mueser, 2003). Substance use, moreover, is not an obstacle to success in competitive employment, presumably because work reinforces sobriety (Sengupta et al., 1998). Supported employment programmes accept and place substance-abusing clients with mental illness as they would any other client.

Integration of vocational rehabilitation and mental health services

Research reveals that better results can be obtained if vocational programmes are an integrated part of a mental health agency or team, rather than being provided by a separate entity. Supported employment programmes are more likely to be successful if vocational staff meet often with clinical case managers and the case managers are involved in the employment effort (Gowdy et al., 2003). In those vocational services that are integrated with the clinical programme, the client dropout rate is lower, communication is better, and clinical information is more likely to find its way into the vocational plan (Drake et al., 2003). The integration of vocational and clinical services facilitates the referral of clients, helps synchronise medication and housing needs with the job, and clarifies the responsibility for follow-up (Bond, 2004a).

Competitive employment is the goal

Supporters of the IPS model contend that most people with serious mental illness can achieve competitive employment and that sheltered work settings are unnecessary. Many observers consider this conclusion to be questionable. If it were true, then the success rate in placing people in competitive work through supported employment would be close to 100%, not 50%. It is true that most of those clients who are working in a sheltered setting would prefer supported competitive employment (Bedell *et al.*, 1998), but the question remains as to whether all can achieve this end. This issue will be discussed in more detail in the next section.

Rapid job search and placement

Research suggests that preparatory work-readiness training does not increase the likelihood of eventual competitive employment and that rapid job placement is more successful. Eight of nine randomised controlled studies demonstrate better work outcomes for clients who embark on rapid job search and placement instead of being offered assessment, skills training and vocational counselling (Bond, 2004a). This is good news for the service agency, as it saves unnecessary expense, and for the service users, the large majority of whom prefer rapid job placement (Bond *et al.*, 1995).

Attention to the mentally ill person's preferences

Job-finding in a supported employment programme is ideally based on the service user's preferences, strengths and previous work experience, rather than on a pool of currently available jobs. Most people with mental illness have specific preferences about the type of work, hours, job location and pay. Matching the person to the job on these criteria results in higher rates of job placement and longer job tenure (Becker *et al.*, 1998). Changes in the service user's preferences, it emerges, are more likely to occur after trying out a job than after vocational counselling, suggesting that job experience is the better approach to selecting the best placement (Becker *et al.*, 1998).

Continuous assessment and support

The most valuable assessment is made *after* the person with mental illness begins working on a job, not before, as occurs in traditional vocational rehabilitation programmes. The employee with mental illness may need support and services for sustained periods of time. One follow-up study of service users, conducted 3.5 years after placement through a supported employment programme, found that sustained employment was nearly three times more likely for those clients who received ongoing support (McHugo *et al.*, 1998). A follow-up study of the conversion of a day-treatment programme to supported employment found that 86% of users were still receiving services ten years later (Salyers *et al.*, 2004).

Supported employment

I've had this job working with dogs for three years. I got it through my job coach. One day I was real upset and I said to my boss, 'I want to quit my job,' and she said, 'Why don't you just take the day off and think about it?' and I came back to work in about a week. So she really helped me.

Personalised benefits planning is part of the package

Job coaches provide help in understanding the complex rules governing disability benefits to assist clients in making the best employment decision. A Vermont study that deployed benefits counsellors to work closely with supported employment programmes throughout the state found that client earnings doubled as a result of the intervention (Tremblay et al., 2004).

There is now a good deal of evidence for the effectiveness of IPS and supported employment, including several randomised controlled trials and a series of studies of the conversion of standard day-care programmes into IPS or supported employment sites (Bond, 2004b). Studies of the effectiveness of converting six New England day programmes to supported employment found similar results at each site (Drake et al., 1994; Drake et al., 1996; Bailey et al., 1998; Gold and Marrone, 1998; Becker et al., 2001). There was a common research design to these day-treatment conversion studies: the day-programme was discontinued, and in its place clients were provided with supported employment services and the day-programme staff were reassigned to other jobs within the agency. The result was a large increase in client employment rates from 13% to 37% at the conversion sites, compared with a non-significant change from 12% to 15% at the control-comparison day-care sites. No negative outcomes, such as relapse and hospital admission, were observed, and consumers, family members and staff all liked the change. The former day-treatment clients spent more time in the community, and the change resulted in cost savings (Bond, 2004a).

Eleven randomised controlled studies of supported employment or IPS conducted in several US states, in which the control groups were usually subjects in traditional vocational services or sheltered employment, have shown substantial advantages in each case for supported employment and IPS. Competitive employment rates in the supported employment and IPS cohorts ranged from 27% to 77% and in the control groups from 6% to 40%. In each study, the rate of competitive employment was never less than double that of the control group, and the difference was sometimes much greater. On average, the rate of competitive employment in the supported employment samples was 60% and in the control groups 21% (Bond, 2004a). In addition to this US research, a British study of supported employment for people recovering from their first episode of psychosis demonstrated an increase in employment from 10% to 41% in the course of a year (Rinaldi *et al.*, 2004).

11.5 Sheltered work: does it have a future?

Sheltered work, or 'industrial therapy', was developed in northern Europe and the USA after the Second World War and was based on work programmes for people disabled by such illnesses as tuberculosis and heart disease. In sheltered workshops, a wide range of semiskilled and low-skilled tasks are performed, frequently for contracts obtained from private industry. Sometimes the work comprises a series of repetitive tasks that would lead to high staff turnover if performed in house by the private company's own employees. Many sheltered workshop employees are paid piece-rate, which means that seriously handicapped workers can be employed, but if their pace of work is slow they may earn below the minimum hourly wage.

Sheltered workshops are no longer popular. Critics argue that people placed in low-demand settings may fail to advance to more challenging work, even though they are capable of doing so (Lehman, 1995). Paid sheltered work, it is argued, may not yield the same non-vocational benefits – such as better control of symptoms, higher self-esteem and improved quality of life – as competitive employment (Bond *et al.*, 2001). When resources are limited, analysts suggest, they are more usefully devoted to supported employment. Supporters of sheltered work point out that for some people with limited functioning capacity, sheltered settings may be the only feasible workplace (Black, 1992). At the Mental Health Center of Boulder County in Colorado, for example, where both supported employment and a modernised sheltered workshop are available, a high rate of employment has been achieved. In 2002, more than half of the working-age adults with psychotic illness were in paid employment, 12% of the group in the sheltered workshop. A reduction in funding of the sheltered workshop in 2003 led to a decrease in employment there to 6% of the adults with psychosis, with no concomitant increase in supported employment. Thus, although it would have been easy for a client to move from the sheltered workshop to supported employment in the Boulder system, and such a move was strongly encouraged, no one in fact was able to manage it when sheltered work became less available. It became apparent that very few of the people employed at the sheltered workshop could hold down a job in the competitive labour market. Many of the workshop employees work slowly and inefficiently at the most routine tasks and require a lot of day-to-day supervision. Without the workshop, overall employment for people with serious mental illness in Boulder would be reduced significantly.

To address some of the critics' concerns, it is possible to redesign the sheltered workshop to be more like the social firms described in the next chapter. This has been done with the sheltered workshop in Boulder, which has been reconfigured as a packaging and mailing business with employees involved in the administration of the business through a management council. Involvement of workers in business planning has the potential to increase the non-vocational benefits of the job. One study of clients in sheltered work demonstrated that the workers' levels of self-esteem were related positively to only one factor – the degree of importance that the worker felt the public ascribed to their job (Dick and Shepherd, 1994). This finding suggests that the more the worker understands the value of the business product to the community, the greater will be his or her psychological wellbeing. The Boulder sheltered work setting has been modernised with new equipment to be more commercially competitive and has also been made more integrated by hiring more mentally healthy workers. The setting is now attractive to the local social services department as a work-training and evaluation option for 'welfare-to-work' clients who have been unemployed for an extended period.

Many commentators argue that an array of vocational opportunities, from sheltered work to supported employment, is in the best interests of the service user (Starks *et al.*, 2000; Krupa, 1998). Vocational workers at Thresholds in Chicago, IL, for example, advocate the enclave model of semi-sheltered group placement of workers in commercial settings in addition to the supported employment model (Shimon and Forman, 1991). The Village, an employment programme in Los Angeles, CA, has developed a menu of employment options for consumers that range from group placements and transitional employment, through temporary jobs in agency-run businesses, to full-time community employment (Chandler *et al.*, 1999).

Behind much of the criticism of sheltered work settings is the cultural emphasis, particularly strong in the USA, on individualism and independence. Just as independent living is assumed to be superior to group homes for people with mental illness, so competitive employment is assumed to be better than sheltered or semi-sheltered work. This philosophical adherence to independence has been challenged, however, by the mental-health organisational theorist James Mandiberg. Mandiberg (1999) argues that many people with mental illness belong to a consumer subculture that offers a number of benefits, including social support and a sense of community. Mandiberg suggests that both work and housing programmes can be developed that build on the mutual support that exists in the consumer subculture. The psychosocial clubhouse model to be discussed in Chapter 14 is an example of this principle. We can appreciate Mandiberg's viewpoint better if we use the analogy of cultural subgroups within a larger mainstream society. We would think it improper to fragment a Chinese-American community and insist that community members disperse their homes around the city and work in mainstream businesses. It may be equally culturally insensitive to insist that people with mental illness should never live and work with other people with mental illness. If, on the other hand, we see a value in building upon the mutual supports to be found in consumer subculture, then we will be more positive about congregate work settings and particularly interested in the employment model to be presented in the next chapter, consumer-employing and consumer-run social firms or affirmative businesses.

11.6 Conclusions

The traditional 'train and place' vocational rehabilitation model, designed originally for people with physical disabilities, has never been effective for people with mental illness. Specialised vocational programmes for people with mental illness became effective in helping clients adjust to paid employment in the 1970s, but it was not until the advent of supported employment in the 1990s that vocational programmes achieved success in maintaining clients in competitive employment. A well-researched refinement of the supported employment approach, individual placement and support (IPS), has a strong evidence base supporting the principles of the approach. These principles include basing eligibility for placement on consumer choice, integrating vocational and clinical services, rapid job placement, and providing ongoing assessment and support. Not everyone with mental illness is capable of competitive employment, and there is still a place for sheltered and semi-sheltered work settings in the spectrum of vocational opportunities for people with mental illness.

Social firms

12.1 Italian cooperatives

Post-war psychiatric deinstitutionalisation got off to a late start in Italy, and, once started, took a rather different path compared with the psychiatric services elsewhere in Western Europe. As the process unfolded, the psychiatric innovators in northern Italy developed a new approach to providing employment to people with mental illness. The innovation is called a social enterprise (*impresa sociale*); alternatively, because it adheres to a business structure commonly found in north-eastern Italy – the worker cooperative – it is often referred to under that name (*cooperativa di lavoro*). The model has been adopted elsewhere (usually without the worker-cooperative business structure), and in English-speaking countries it has come to be called a social firm or, as in North America, an affirmative business. The social firm is a business with a dual mission: it is established to create employment for people with disabilities and to provide a useful product or service. The company often employs a mixture of disabled and non-disabled employees in a roughly 50:50 proportion. It is worth telling the story of the development of this innovation in some detail.

In 1961, a young Italian psychiatrist, Franco Basaglia, took over the director-ship of an asylum in Gorizia near the then Yugoslavian border. Working with a small group of associates, he gradually eliminated the use of restraints, straitjackets, bars and keys and restored personal clothing and dignity to the inmates, as many had done elsewhere in Europe. In due course, Basaglia's assistants took positions at other asylums across Italy, where they replicated the process. In 1971, Basaglia moved to manage the San Giovanni Hospital in Trieste, where he and his associates developed a showcase of what alternative psychiatry could accomplish. Patients were transferred to mixed-gender wards, and many were subsequently released or given 'guest' (*ospite*) status, so that they could come and go from the hospital at will. Community teams were established to work with patients and their families in different sectors of the city and surrounding country. The debate on the place of the asylum and the person with mental illness in society was picked up by newspapers, radio and television. Basaglia did not shy away from this public exposure but rather used it to advance his mission. To draw townspeople on to the asylum grounds, the hospital sponsored film festivals, art exhibitions, concerts and theatre productions. In 1973, a group of artists, staff and patients constructed a huge blue horse, Marco Cavallo, representing the animal that used to cart away the hospital's dirty linen. Patients used to quip that the carthorse was the only creature that ever escaped the institution. In a gesture reminiscent of the Trojan horse, the belly of the statue was filled with letters from patients expressing their aspirations for the future, and the horse was drawn in procession by hospital residents and workers through the asylum gates and down to the centre of town. Several hundred patients joined the procession and, some for the first time, went around the town celebrating their newfound freedom (Dell'Acqua and Dezza, 1985; Scheper-Hughes and Lovell, 1987; Donnelly, 1992).

The story of the Trieste experience is of interest for a couple of reasons. Basaglia's willingness to get involved in a public debate about the future of people with mental illness stands in contrast to the usual practice of managers of mental health services and helps us understand how the Trieste team was able to go further in setting up work opportunities for people with serious mental illness. The first worker cooperative for ex-patients was developed in 1973 as a reaction to work therapy, which the Trieste team considered exploitative. The patients were given the rights of both workers and business owners. The first cooperative provided employment in cleaning and maintaining public buildings, and by 1985 it was employing 130 workers (Dell'Acqua and Dezza, 1985; Mosher and Burti, 1989). As more cooperatives were developed, the managers involved the local trade unions in their plans. By 1994, the consortium of cooperatives in Trieste had grown to impressive dimensions, with an annual turnover of £2.6 million (US$5 million), and included a hotel, a café, a restaurant, a transportation business and a building-renovation company. The consortium employed a mixed workforce of mentally disabled and healthy workers in manufacturing and service enterprises (Warner, 2004). According to the figures for 2004, the total annual income of the network of cooperatives established by the Trieste mental health service had grown to €10.7 million (at that time, £7.3 million or US$14 million). At the time of writing most of the original firms continue in operation, new ones have been developed, and a number of independent social cooperatives have also been set up by non-governmental agencies. The Hotel Tritone, one of the original businesses, has proven particularly successful. The opening of a second hotel is planned, and a franchising venture is in the works. The cleaning sector has expanded considerably, and now all of the office- and street-cleaning contracts for the municipality of Trieste have been won by social firms. Other products and services include shopping for the homebound, landscaping and bookbinding. About 300 disadvantaged and disabled people are employed in the Trieste co-operatives, approximately half of whom are people with mental illness. In addition, about 180 people with mental illness have training positions in the cooperatives reimbursed by a governmental stipend (*borsa lavoro*).

The social firm approach has been replicated in many other parts of Italy. In nearby Pordenone, the enterprises include those offering cleaning, making park furniture, nursing-home aides and home help for disabled people. In Palmanova, a broad array of cooperatives have been developed, including restaurants, a horticultural nursery and several tourist hotels, in which some of the consumer employees live rent-free (Warner, 2004). In Rome, there are around 30 cooperatives, with products and services that include graphics and printing and a laundry; these businesses employ 450 people, more than half of whom are disabled. Turin has an extensive network of social firms, including gardening and catering. There are fewer cooperatives in the south of Italy, but some can be found in such towns as Reggio Calabria and Bari (www.cefec.org). By 1997, there were about 1600 social cooperatives throughout Italy, employing around 40 000 workers, 40% of whom were disabled, and with an annual turnover of €590 million (at that time , US$770 million, £400 million) (Schwarz and Higgins, 1999). The proportion of these disabled workers who have mental illness is, however, unknown.

The Italian social cooperatives, according to statute, are categorized as type A and type B. Type A enterprises provide public services, such as youth centres and home-health services, or operate educational programmes like libraries and health-worker training. Type B cooperatives develop work opportunities, such as factories and farms, for people with social handicaps and disabilities, e.g. ex-prisoners, substance abusers and people with psychiatric and physical disabilities. The category that concerns us here is the type B cooperative. Some small and some large, type B enterprises compete successfully with local businesses, selling their products and services on the open marketplace or winning contracts by competitive bids. In Pordenone and Trieste, about 90% of the work contracts are made with public agencies such as the municipality, hospitals, schools and fire stations. Initially, the Trieste cooperatives used a significant public subsidy. In 1994, direct grants, donated space and staff time contributed by the mental health service amounted to about 20% of the total budget, but by 2004, the subsidy had dropped to almost zero. The Pordenone cooperatives have always operated with a negligible subsidy. In each consortium, about half of the regular workers are mentally ill or are otherwise disabled, earning a standard full-time wage. Some mentally ill people work part-time as trainees and receive a training stipend (*borsa lavoro*). In Trieste, people receiving the training stipend graduate in significant numbers each year to full employment within the cooperative, but some less productive workers may remain on the *borsa* for years. Unlike most US programmes for people with mental illness, the Italian cooperatives advertise widely and have high community visibility. Thus, the scale and social impact of these enterprises exceed the usual achievements of vocational programmes (Savio and Righetti, 1993; Warner, 2004).

A support organisation for social cooperatives, the Consorzio per l'impresa sociale, was founded in north-eastern Italy in 1996. This provides direct services, such as accounting, legal advice, business and market planning and training, to developing social enterprises. It has also launched a number of community initiatives, including franchising successful business, the development of a transnational network of social firms, assisting in the development of social cooperatives in neighbouring Slovenia and elsewhere, and establishing a national media relations network (Schwarz and Higgins, 1999).

12.2 What is a social firm?

The social firm model has been adopted with more or less success in a variety of countries around the world. As the model has diffused, the accepted principles of these enterprises have been defined as follows. A social firm:

- is created to offer employment to people with a disability or a labour-market disadvantage, and a substantial proportion of its employees (over a third) will fit this description;
- produces goods and services to pursue its social mission;
- pays every worker a market wage appropriate to the job, regardless of the worker's productive capacity;
- establishes the same rights, opportunities and obligations for all employees;
- creates an empowering atmosphere for workers and provides reasonable accommodations for disabled workers' needs;
- is a viable concern operating in the open market.

The social firm may get additional income for vocational training, but until it has freed itself from other subsidies such as start-up grants, it may be referred to as an 'emerging' social firm (Schwarz and Higgins, 1999).

12.3 Social firms around the world

Since the mid 1990s, there has been a distinct increase in interest in social firms as a vocational model, partly as a consequence of the development of support structures in Italy and elsewhere that have fostered transfer of technology. Also since that time, businesses of this type have operated in Germany, Britain, Switzerland, Ireland, Austria, Spain, Japan, New Zealand, Australia, the USA and several other countries. A survey conducted in 1999 concluded that there were about 2000 social firms in Europe, employing approximately 47 000 workers, 40–50% of whom were disabled (Schwarz and Higgins, 1999).

Germany

Outside Italy, the country with largest number of social firms is Germany. In 1999, Germany had approximately 300 such companies (*Integrationsfirmen*), with a combined workforce of 6000, 50% of whom were disabled. The first enterprises were founded in 1978, and their numbers have been growing since. German social firms generally are not run as worker cooperatives, but efforts have been made to create partnerships between workers and management. The main objective of these enterprises is to provide permanent full-wage work for people with psychiatric disabilities. These non-profit companies are usually specialised firms producing foods (often health foods) or technical products, providing domestic services, such as moving, painting and repairs, and offering office services and printing. Commonly, about 30% of the company's net income is derived from government reimbursement in the form of wage supplements that are awarded for each disabled worker at a diminishing rate over three years. Unless new disabled workers are hired, subsidies dwindle, until the company has to survive on earnings alone. With careful planning, this is feasible, and only a small number of the social enterprises established in Germany have been forced to shut down (Stastny *et al.*, 1992; Schwarz and Higgins, 1999).

The German social enterprise movement is supported by a national non-profit agency, Fachberatung fuer Arbeits und Firmenprojekte (FAF), which was launched in the late 1980s and now represents about 200 social firms. FAF provides business consulting, training for social firm managers and other technical support, and has attained a high level of recognition with the federal government (Schwarz and Higgins, 1999).

Britain

The number of social firms in Britain before 1997 was just six. Since then, a national support group, Social Firms UK, has fostered the development of many more of these enterprises, so that the number at the time of writing is over 70. Technical assistance provided by the Italian and German support organisations has played a large part in the growth of the British social firm movement. By 1999, the British companies were providing employment for about 400 people, a third of whom were disabled. About a third of the firms are worker-cooperatives. The British social firms are, or aim to be, sustainable businesses without a public subsidy. Some of the emerging firms still require a subsidy or are not yet able to pay disabled workers a wage that exceeds social security benefits (Schwarz and Higgins, 1999). Social Firms UK has established a franchising operation for some of the more successful businesses, including a soap-manufacturing and retail venture, an aquarium-maintenance business, a coffee shop, a hotel, a home health aide service, a computer-recycling company and a drive-through laundry (see www.socialfirms.co.uk).

Ireland

The importance of business viability is illustrated by the story of Irish Social Firms in Dublin. In the 1990s, this consortium operated a restaurant, a lunch counter, a wool shop and a retail furniture store, staffed by people with mental illness, but these businesses have all been closed down in recent years due to the size of the subsidy required to sustain the businesses.

Japan

Social firms have proven viable in Japan. In Obihiro in northern Japan consumer-employing businesses include a vegetable farm, a coffee shop and a hotel kitchen. In Okayama, mentally ill workers provide milk delivery to 250 households, operate a meals-on-wheels service and run a café. The Japanese social firm model, based on the Italian approach, has proven possible because of the recently liberalised access for grass-roots organisations to achieve non-profit corporate status, which brings with it commercial advantages in such areas as the rental of office space (J. Mandiberg, personal communication, 2003).

New Zealand and Australia

Workwise in New Zealand operates a number of social firms, including Hamlin Road Farms in Counties Manukau, south of Auckland, where the products include free-range eggs, organic watercress, flowers and vegetables. The farm employs around 20 workers, many of whom are people with serious mental illnesses who are not ready for competitive employment. Other successful enterprises include a soap factory and a handmade toy production company. The economic boom in New Zealand, with accompanying full employment, has increased government interest in sponsoring vocational models for people with disabilities, including social firms and supported education.

Social Firms Australia has opened a supermarket and is preparing to open several other businesses, including a carwash café. In both Australia and New Zealand, a common pattern of social firm development is to open a franchise of a successful company, including some of the franchise opportunities offered by Social Firms UK.

The Netherlands, Greece, Spain and Austria

There are 20 to 30 projects operating in the Netherlands as social firms. These firms were developed by psychiatric service organisations and receive funding from the state and health insurance. A national social firm support organisation, CEFEC Netherlands, provides loans, consultation and business planning assistance to the emerging businesses. In Greece, there are about 20 social cooperatives, several of which are primarily serving people with psychiatric disabilities. The European Union has provided substantial support to the Greek ventures, and a national association, the Pan-Hellenic Union for Psychosocial Rehabilitation and Work Integration, launched in 1994, has helped support the growth of the social firm model. Pro Mente Kärnten in Carinthia in Austria runs four social firms, in which wages are subsidised by the government departments of labour and disability and by the local authority. In Andalusia in Spain in 1999, there were eight social firms employing 340 workers, half of whom were disabled. The Spanish enterprises are supported by Iniciativas de Empleo Andaluzas (IDEA), founded in 1991 and based in Seville (Schwarz and Higgins, 1999).

Canada

Virtually all of the vocational programming for mentally ill people in Toronto, Canada, has been converted to the social enterprise model. In Canada, social firms are generally referred to as 'affirmative businesses', but when they are controlled and operated by service users or consumers they are termed 'alternative businesses'. One such programme is a consumer-run courier business, A-Way Express, which was launched in 1987 and operates city-wide. The employees and managers are all people with mental illness. The couriers use the public transportation system to pick up and deliver packages across the city, communicating with their dispatch office by walkie-talkie (Hartl, 1992). Such consumer-controlled businesses are particularly empowering, since they offer the opportunity for workers to become involved in a variety of tasks and responsibilities and the potential for advancement within the enterprise, even though the individual's day-to-day work may be fairly routine (Krupa, 1998). The Ontario Council of Alternative Businesses represents 11 other consumer-run firms in Ontario that employ 600 people with psychiatric disabilities. There are three such enterprises in Toronto: the Raging Spoon Café, the Inspirations/Ideas studio space and New Look Cleaning (www.icomm.ca/ocab). Another social firm that has been operating in Toronto since the late 1980s is a cleaning and maintenance service called Fresh Start. The social firm movement has not taken off with as much vigour in the other Canadian provinces, and there are no completely consumer-operated alternative businesses outside Ontario (J. Trainor, personal communication, 2005).

The USA

There are some successful examples of social firms ('affirmative businesses') in the USA. Monadnock Family Services in Keene, NH, has established a cooperative with projects that began by buying, renovating and selling houses and has now moved on to building garden furniture (Boyles, 1988; F. Silvestri, Personal Communication, 2005). An Asian-American mental health clinic in Washington state established a successful consumer-run espresso bar in 1995 (Kakutani, 1998). Minnesota Diversified Industries (MDI), founded in 1968, is a non-profit business employing more than 1000 people that provides packaging and distribution services and manufactures plastic products. Aspen Diversified Industries (ADI), based in Colorado Springs, is an enterprise offering mainly janitorial, warehousing and assembly services that contracts with Colorado mental health centres to provide rehabilitation and employment opportunities for their clients.

Some of MDI's and ADI's most lucrative contracts have come through a national agency, the National Industries for the Severely Handicapped (NISH). This entity is designated by the federal government to facilitate the purchase of products and services for governmental agencies from non-profit businesses that employ people with disabilities. NISH is a product of the Javits-Wagner-O'Day (JWOD) Act, which was passed in 1971 to increase employment for people with severe disabilities. The JWOD programme works with over 600 non-profit agencies across the USA to provide employment to 36 000 Americans with disabilities, a proportion of whom suffer from mental illness (www.jwod.gov).

Although there are support organisations for affirmative businesses in the USA, such as the Affirmative Business Alliance of North America and Workability Americas, the model has not achieved as much prominence or vitality as it has in parts of Europe, in Ontario and in New Zealand. Some of the older and larger North American affirmative businesses are, in fact, modified sheltered workshops and did not develop out of the European concept (Krupa, 1998). In part, the slow growth of the US movement is due to the existence of a competing model – the supported employment approach described in the previous chapter, which has become disseminated quite widely in the USA since the mid 1990s, achieving success in placing people with mental illness in competitive employment. Consequently, it is more common to find consumer-employing businesses being offered as part of a spectrum of vocational services that includes supported employment. This is the case in Los Angeles, CA, where the Village Integrated Service Agency offers its clients a menu of vocational opportunities, on which are listed five businesses run by the agency. These enterprises are a maintenance business, clerical services, an 85-seat delicatessan, a banking service for people with mental illness and a convenience store (Chandler et al., 1999). The mental health service in Boulder, Colorado, has also taken a menu approach, with results that will be described in the next chapter.

12.4 Recipes for success

In parts of northern Italy, social enterprises have established themselves in the open market, becoming viable not only as a rehabilitation model but also as an important part of the local economy. In other places, including large parts of Italy, the number of people employed through social firms is still small. Can this model become a dominant rehabilitation paradigm anywhere but Italy? Realistically, it seems somewhat perverse that in order to find employment for people with mental illness, we should have to develop entire business enterprises to do so, especially since the problems in creating and operating a new business are legion. It seems there would have to be some special factors militating for the success of social firms. What might these be?

Government policies and statutes favouring disabled people seem to be critical. In Italy, legislation offers tax advantages to worker cooperatives and funding to social enterprises. In Korea, laws require businesses to employ disabled people or to contribute funds for their employment elsewhere. In Germany, government provides wage supplements to new disabled employees of social firms. And in the USA, JWOD legislation directs government entities to use the products and services of social firms. The legislative possibilities are numerous, but they all address a critical issue: how to make an accommodation for the business disadvantage of employing less productive workers.

Social firms may also achieve success by finding the right market niche. Many such enterprises, for example, have gained a market edge by competing for contracts with public agencies. Such agencies (for example, hospitals) often have a special concern about the social exclusion of disabled people or have a strategic need to be seen to be serving the public interest. There may also be practical advantages. The cleaning businesses in Pordenone, Italy, for example, were successful in obtaining contracts with public facilities in part because the unionised workforce previously doing the work was relatively expensive and inefficient. The market niche may come from the special qualities of the workers. It is not easy, for example, to find people who are willing to work as home health aides, but people who themselves have disabilities may find this work acceptable and be able to call upon unusual reserves of empathy and patience.

The public orientation of the social firm network may also help the firm to earn contracts through a willingness to help solve community problems. Managers from a group of cooperatives in Trieste, Italy, for example, met with city officials about existing community problems. In discussing ways to clean up a run-down section of the city, it became apparent that one significant problem was the number of abandoned broken-down motor scooters littering the streets. This observation led to a plan to develop a scooter-salvaging workshop, staffed by young disadvantaged people, many of whom had a history of disassembling scooters on the street in order to steal parts. Another partnership between the public need and the social cooperatives in Trieste resulted in an operation that provides comprehensive long-term management and repair for public buildings coupled with moving services, in an approach that minimises public-sector management expense.

In the next chapter, we will look at how the consumption market of people with mental illness themselves may create special opportunities for consumer-employing businesses.

Social firms naturally seek out labour-intensive production processes in order to maximise employment prospects with the least capital investment. As a result, they may gravitate towards cleaning and repair services; handmade products, like wooden toys; organic food production that is not driven by large investments in agricultural machinery and fertiliser; carwashes; and bicycle-repair shops. On the other hand, a consortium of social firms may choose to develop a business that is profitable but employs relatively few disabled people in order to use the earnings of this enterprise to offset the losses of others. Such tension between the dual missions of the entity is unavoidable. Social firm managers in Trieste and elsewhere emphasise the need to maintain a diversified source of revenue from a range of different services and products. Social enterprises are often small and try to offer a range of services and products in order to be adaptable to changing market circumstances and to provide a range of work opportunities. Boring and repetitive tasks are avoided as far as possible and there is an emphasis on producing a high-quality product in a high-quality work environment (Grove *et al.*, 1997).

A factor that has helped advance the social firm model for people with mental illness is the general lack, until the 1990s, of adequate vocational rehabilitation alternatives. Now that the supported employment model, individual placement and support (IPS), has been shown to be effective and is being tested and promoted outside the USA, it will be interesting to see whether social firms hold their own. In fact, social firms may continue to be attractive, despite the competition with supported employment, because the approach fits well with the interest in the recovery model and in service-user empowerment (see Chapter 14). There are few better indications of recovery than returning to work and little that could better demonstrate empowerment than gaining control over the direction of one's workplace. One of the reasons for the success of alternative businesses in Toronto, for example, is the long-standing strength of the consumer movement in that city (Krupa, 1998). Social firms provide a greater opportunity for consumer-worker solidarity and the development of a sense of community than does the placement of workers in individual supported employment slots. One manager of a set of social firms in Trieste described this sense of community in the workforce as '*una piccola famiglia allargata*' – a small extended family. In the worker-cooperative setting, this sense of community can become quite altruistic, such as when workers in a Trieste social firm choose to renounce their annual bonus or some of their annual vacation in order to help the firm's bottom line. As another Trieste social cooperative manager put it, 'We are not just producing economic capital, but social capital.' There appears to be no reason that social firms and supported employment cannot operate side by side in the same rehabilitation system. In Trieste, which is rich in social firms, rehabilitation workers also place people with mental illness in jobs in small private businesses and support them long-term, much as a supported employment job coach does. As mentioned, similar mixed systems operate in Los Angeles and Boulder.

Social firm managers emphasise the importance of having strong links between the psychiatric care system and the employment setting. Consumer-employing businesses cannot be developed in a vacuum. A successful business can be established only if there are capable people in the consumer pool whose illnesses are stabilised with adequate psychiatric care. Ongoing support for the consumer-worker, moreover, requires close working relationships between the social firm manager (the employer) and the clinical staff, as is the case also with supported employment. It is for this reason, among others, that the managers of Italian social cooperatives emphasise that such enterprises as these can be developed only with the collaboration of a superior psychiatric care system.

It seems clear that the creation of support entities has helped the dissemination of social firms in those regions where they have become successful. Support bodies, such as IDEA in Spain, facilitate the transfer of technology, providing business consulting, training for managers and other assistance. New businesses often need help with business-plan development, market research and locating start-up funding, and they can usually find that technical support through local small-business development agencies. The unusual nature of social firms, however, makes it more difficult for these enterprises to obtain such assistance locally. The training of social firm managers is a particularly important issue, since individuals with entrepreneurial skills are unlikely to have the knowledge and ability to work with people with psychiatric disabilities, and vice versa. Other technical services that the support network can provide are the development of promotional materials, directories and technical guides (Grove *et al.*, 1997).

Support networks are valuable in developing linkages between social firms, other businesses and legislators. FAF in Germany, for example, works closely with the Department of Labour and Social Affairs in developing and monitoring social firms. International training seminars have been organised with the help of the Confederation of European Firms, Employment Initiatives and Cooperatives (CEFEC). The support network can also collect and disseminate information about social enterprises and can lobby policymakers to sponsor legislation advantageous to businesses employing disabled people.

12.5 Conclusions

The social firm model was developed in north-eastern Italy in the 1970s and has become increasingly successful in several parts of the world. Across Europe, there is growing interest in the approach as an alternative to the standard 'train and place' form of vocational rehabilitation. We have argued that the ideal vocational rehabilitation system will be one that provides a spectrum of opportunities from sheltered to independent. Social firms offer a more sheltered alternative to continuous supported employment, and enterprises that involve workers in management are more empowering. They may, therefore, offer a good choice of permanent employment or transitional employment to many people with mental illness. German research indicates that about a third of those who leave employment with a social firm find a job in the open market (Schwarz and Higgins, 1999), suggesting that these enterprises may be quite efficient as transitional employment programmes. Social firms enhance the spectrum of work opportunities, helping to expand the choices available to those who would like to work, and making the opportunities as normalising and as genuinely integrated into mainstream life of the community as is compatible with job tenure and job satisfaction.

Innovative strategies

13.1 An economic development approach

A number of innovative strategies that call for new perspectives on the issue of social integration have proven valuable in helping people with mental illness reach for full citizenship in society. One of these strategies is the economic development approach, which posits that people with mental illness wield economic power that can be turned to their advantage, in terms of both creating employment opportunities and improving their social and financial welfare.

Psychiatrist Paul Polak developed a model community support system for people with serious mental illness in southwest Denver, Colorado, in the 1970s. Polak left that position in 1980 to found a non-profit developing world development company, International Development Enterprises, which has enjoyed success in creating grass-roots income-producing opportunities for poor people in the developing world. Polak's work, which led to his being picked by *Scientific American* in 2004 as the top contributor to global agricultural policy, is based on a concise formulation of principles for designing effective development projects, namely:

- Evaluate the day-to-day economy of the disadvantaged group and the effect of economic incentives.
- Identify areas of the group members' production or consumption that might provide income-generating opportunities. For example, give ownership to poor people of an expensive fraction of their consumption, such as transportation.
- Focus on a single area that will leverage changes in several other domains of daily economic life.
- Market the innovation assertively to ensure broad availability.

Like poor farmers in the developing world, people with serious mental illness in the West are an economically disadvantaged group with reservoirs of untapped productive capacity. One of the authors (RW) and Paul Polak examined whether the economic development approach that was effective with developing world disadvantaged populations could be useful in advancing the employment and economic conditions of people with mental illness in the developed world. The goal was to develop consumer-employing businesses that would exploit the purchasing power of people with mental illness. Such an approach has the merit of recirculating money through the community to create an economic multiplier effect, equivalent to establishing local ownership of the ghetto grocery store so that outside owners do not drain capital from the neighbourhood. To pursue this goal, in 1992 we interviewed 50 mentally ill people living in Boulder, Colorado, to learn about their personal finances and to spot potential money-making opportunities. Eighteen of our subjects were unemployed, 18 were part-time employed, five were employed full-time and three had an independent source of income. We asked them about their:

- cash income, from working or from disability benefits;
- non-cash income, such as goods and services provided to them, including psychiatric care, free medication and housing.

We calculated a cash value of these goods and services.

We also asked about their:

- cash expenses;
- non-cash expenses.

This latter component refers to goods and services that the subject provided in exchange for cash or other goods and services. An example would be letting someone stay in one's apartment in exchange for food, protection or some other benefit. Again, we calculated a cash value for the exchange.

We found the average monthly income and expenses to be as follows:

- Cash income: US$774
- Non-cash income: US$1405
- Cash expenses: US$704
- Non-cash expenses: US$86

The total consumption market of the people in our survey was the combination of their cash expenses (what they spent, US$704) and the non-cash income of goods and services (what they were provided, US$1405). Thus, it was apparent that the consumers controlled some sizeable markets – over US$2000 a month (£1300 in 1992), in various goods and services. The monthly figures for the top six areas of consumption were as follows:

- Psychiatric treatment: US$1116
- Rent: US$295
- Food: US$108
- Medication: US$90
- Transportation: US$83
- Meals out: US$71

After reviewing these data, we suggested that a number of consumer-employing enterprises could be developed that would serve people with mental illness and exploit their consumption markets. They included: (i) treatment-related services for people with mental illness, (ii) a housing cooperative, (iii) a food cooperative, (iv) a consumer-oriented pharmacy, (v) a cafeteria and (vi) transportation services (Warner and Polak, 1995). We will discuss here three of these options that have proven to be valuable sources of employment and/or economic advancement for people with mental illness: (i) employing people with mental illness in the psychiatric service system, (ii) a consumer-oriented, consumer-employing pharmacy and (iii) housing cooperatives.

13.2 Employing consumers in the psychiatric service system

A group based in Denver, Colorado, the Regional Assessment and Training Center, has developed a programme to train people with serious mental illness to become case-manager aides, residential facility staff members and job coaches in the mental health centres across the state. In operation since 1986, the programme enrols its trainees – people who have made good recovery from serious mental illness – in six weeks of classroom education and then places them in on-the-job internships for three months, working on treatment teams for people with mental illness. Programme graduates are hired throughout the mental health system at standard rates of pay. As case-manager aides, they help their clients with a variety of tasks, such as applying for welfare entitlements and finding housing, and counsel them around treatment, work, and issues of day-to day living (Sherman and Porter, 1991). Since the programme's inception, well over 100 consumer mental health workers have been placed in employment throughout the service system, providing models for patients and staff alike of successful recovery from mental illness. Two-thirds of the trainees continue to be employed successfully in the mental health system two years after graduation from the training programme. The programme has been replicated in several other cities and states across the USA, including Washington, DC, Houston, Texas, Utah and Oregon.

In many mental health services, increasing numbers of consumers are being employed in a variety of roles. Around 10% of the workforce of the Pathfinder Trust in London comprises people with mental illness. There is a user-managed employment programme at Southwest London and St George's Mental Health Trust that has been running since the mid 1990s. The senior employment specialist acting as the team coordinator at the time of writing is a user. She describes the work of the team as follows (Harding, 2005):

> **Working as a consumer case-manager aide**
>
> I get to use different skills – composing letters, writing, editing. I get to do research. I get to apply my new skills of teaching and guiding and connecting, always connecting with people, whether they're co-workers or clients. I'm happiest when I'm showing a new client a way, or helping them find a way, because it's more like brainstorming. 'OK, what are we going to do?' 'I'll do some, you do some.' With them taking some responsibility and me taking some responsibility we've connected, bonded in a way. I'm invested in their success, and they get to know me because I'm open and honest about where I've been.

There is a triad of support available . . . enabling people to get jobs by providing weekly details of vacancies and assistance with application forms and interview skills. We then help people to navigate the often tortuous journey between a successful interview and the first day at work by offering benefits advice and information . . . Maintaining confidence is also a large part of the job we do. Finally we offer ongoing support for as long as an individual requires it to enable people to sustain their employment.

At the Mental Health Center of Boulder County, in Colorado, consumers are employed as therapists, case-manager aides, residential counsellors, job coaches, psychosocial clubhouse staff, office workers, consumer organisers and research interviewers. Other mental health agencies have also found the position of peer research interviewer to be one that can be filled successfully by a consumer even when he or she suffers from persistent psychotic symptoms (Lecomte, Cyr *et al.*, 1999). Many mental health agencies hire people with mental illness to be members of a speakers' bureau, teaching about mental illness in schools and community groups (see section 7.6). Increasingly, the experience of having coped with a serious mental illness comes to be seen as a hiring advantage, similar to being bilingual. At the Mental Health Center of Boulder County, most of the entry-level job announcements are posted in the lobby of the agency's offices, and clients are encouraged to apply.

> **Working as a consumer residential aide**
>
> I used to work for one of the residences. I was an overnight counsellor and I had free room and board and I got a stipend cheque every two weeks. I made sure the house was locked up every night, and I let people in when they locked themselves out, and I gave them medications when needed. But even then, I was still isolating myself and hanging out in my room wearing my earplugs to keep the voices away.

A mental health agency can also shift services that are currently contracted to outside enterprises, such as courier services and transcription of dictated medical records, to a consumer enterprise. Janitorial and cleaning services are often thought of in this context, but these jobs are not popular with many mentally ill people. More clients, especially men, are interested in construction and property-repair jobs such as plumbing, wiring, painting and carpentry. In a survey conducted at the mental health centre in Boulder, less than a quarter of the male clients expressed an interest in janitorial work, but more than a third were interested in property repair. Consequently, in 1993 the agency started a small property-repair business employing a non-disabled foreman and a number of part-time consumer workers. The business took over the property maintenance, which previously cost the agency US$30000 (£20000 at that time) a year. It has since expanded and is saving the agency money.

Most of the frequently voiced fears about hiring consumers are not difficult to overcome. Client confidentiality is not an issue if consumer staff are held to the same professional expectations as other staff and are given appropriate training. The consumer's job performance should be separated completely from his or her treatment. Preferably, the consumer staff-person will get treatment at a location that is separate from the work site. This is not always possible in small agencies or in rural locations, but at the very least the job supervisor should not be the same person as the worker's treatment provider. Consumer staff treatment records should be kept in a separate locked filing cabinet, and treatment information should not be used by the job supervisor. Consumer staff should be held by the supervisor to the same job standards as other staff, and the consumer staff-person should not use the work supervisor or co-workers for treatment or expect more on-the-job support and counselling than other workers receive.

Some problems are more difficult. It is not always clear, for example, what allowances should be made on the issue of professional boundaries between staff and clients. Ordinarily, mental health supervisors would insist that professional staff do not enter into sexual, business or certain kinds of social relationships with clients, because the staff-member's power and influence could create the possibility of exploitation. When the consumer staff-member's social group, however, consists in large part of clients of the agency, such a hard and fast rule is not possible. Many of these supervisory issues have to be worked out individually, adhering to the principles that any possibility of client exploitation must be avoided but accepting that the consumer worker cannot be expected to abandon his or her social support system. One of the difficulties that consumer staff-members encounter is a sense of isolation and of being different from their co-workers; so, the importance of in-group support between consumers and consumer-staff should not be underestimated.

Involving and employing consumers at every level of the mental health service system reduces the gulf between 'us' and 'them', enhances respect towards those who are afflicted by illness, and makes clear to clients and staff alike that the goal of treatment is recovery and full participation in society and that the treatment process is not a one-way service relationship with a built-in implication of unbalanced power.

13.3 A consumer-oriented pharmacy

In 1992, a consumer-oriented pharmacy was opened at the Mental Health Center of Boulder County, with the specific intent of providing employment and other benefits to the agency's clients. The original idea to launch such a pharmacy came from James Mandiberg, a social worker and organisational theorist on the faculty of Columbia University in New York City. Profits from the Boulder pharmacy, which amount to nearly US$200 000 (£105 000) a year, are used to support other rehabilitation programmes of the agency. The pharmacy brings a number of benefits. Four consumers are employed as pharmacy technicians alongside three pharmacists. Medication prices are lower than elsewhere in the area. Customers and staff receive more education from the pharmacist on the effects of medication than they would from a high-street retail pharmacy. And pharmacy services are much better coordinated with treatment services than they were previously.

Because of the success of the consumer-oriented pharmacy, the model is being franchised. Other mental health agencies have been invited to establish similar consumer-employing pharmacies under a partnership agreement that specifies that the enterprise will be co-owned and profits divided 50:50 for the first three years of operation, after which the pharmacy will be owned outright by the partner agency. The first replication pharmacy opened in an area west of Denver, Colorado, in 2005.

13.4 Cooperatively owned housing

When mentally ill people become property owners instead of tenants, they achieve a degree of social and economic advancement. Housing cooperatives provide a mechanism for poor people to own their accommodation and offer a number of additional advantages. Such cooperatives not only provide long-term affordable housing but also create a better quality of life for residents, particularly those with special needs, by developing a feeling of community. They build leadership skills among members of the cooperative through the financial, main-tenance and managerial tasks required for the operation of the housing, and they sometimes create opportunities for employment (Davis and Thompson, 1992).

There are, however, relatively few successful examples of cooperative home-ownership by people with mental illness, for a variety of reasons. Mortgage lenders and potential residents may be put off by the cooperative governance structure. Mentally ill people tend to be a fairly mobile group with little capital or monthly income. If hospitalised for a prolonged period, the person may lose benefits and be unable to pay the monthly assessment. In the USA, recipients of supplemental security income (SSI) cannot accumulate capital to purchase housing without adversely affecting their eligibility for benefits. One attempt to create a housing association in which mentally ill people participated in a limited equity housing agreement, the Newell Street Cooperative in Pittsfield, Massachusetts, ended in failure. The project obtained a waiver that allowed governmental rent subsidies to be applied to the purchase of a four-apartment building; when the rent subsidy programme was trimmed, however, the cooperative collapsed. During the one-year period that the cooperative was in operation, improvements were noted in the participants' management skills, self-esteem and sense of mastery.

Despite the difficulties, housing cooperatives for mentally ill people can be viable. Some chapters of the National Alliance for the Mentally Ill (a US organisation of relatives and friends of people with mental illness) have established non-profit housing trusts. The residents of these housing projects are usually mentally ill relatives of the investors. A trust of this type can establish small homes or large apartment complexes and can contract with a local mental health agency to provide appropriate services on premises.

Cooperative housing projects, whether the tenants are owners or not, can become sources of consumer/tenant employment. The Center for Urban Community Services, founded on the Upper West Side of Manhattan by Columbia University, offers supportive housing for mentally ill and mentally healthy poor people at a number of locations. In this project, a private non-profit housing corporation owns the apartment buildings, the mental health agency provides treatment and case management to all the tenants, and a board composed of residents, mental health staff and representatives of the landlord manages the day-to-day operations. Some tenants are given paid jobs on the 24-hours-a-day tenant patrols that provide security and assistance to the residents of the different buildings.

A residential programme in California – the clustered apartment project of the Santa Clara County Mental Health Center – was designed to build community strength among clients living in agency-owned apartments clustered together in a number of different neighbourhoods. Residential staff were encouraged to abandon traditional roles and to become, instead, community organisers. In one programme, all of the staff were consumer-employees. In another, community members provided respite care in a crisis apartment to members who were acutely disturbed. All were successful in building a sense of empowerment among the residents (Mandiberg, 1995).

13.5 An incubator for consumer-run businesses

An alternative to the economic development approach, which focuses on finding a market niche for a consumer-employing business within the consumers' own consumption, is the business incubator approach, which takes the consumers' skills and business interest as the starting point. Business incubation is a commonly used business-development tool. Introduced initially in the declining economy of the post-war 'rustbelt' in the north-eastern USA, this tool is now often used in academic settings, where it provides professionals and scientists with the information, education, advocacy and networking resources necessary to launch new enterprises based on their business ideas. Some business incubators have been established to assist specific target groups such as women entrepreneurs and welfare recipients. Only recently has anyone thought of using this approach to help people with mental illness to launch profitable enterprises. A group of consumers and mental health professionals in Madison, Wisconsin, including James Mandiberg, has done just that.

The Madison-based business incubator, called Enterprise People, consists of a board of consumers, businesspeople and mental health professionals. Over half of the board members are service users. A consumer with a business idea can bring it to the board for discussion and obtain funding for initial training in business skills. The board helps the potential entrepreneur formulate his or her business plan and locate start-up capital. Among the successful enterprises that the incubator has spawned are a small-press publisher of consumer-oriented pamphlets, a gardening and lawn-care operation, a pet-sitting business and a guide-dog-training business. It has also helped a number of individual visual artists develop markets for their work. Many of the consumer entrepreneurs continue to rely on their disability benefits while the business is developing, which allows them to plough back all the profits into the business and avoid any tax liability initially. Since the Madison business incubator for mental health consumers was launched, others have been established in New York and California.

13.6 Conclusions

To develop successful consumer-employing opportunities, it helps to be innovative. Two novel approaches are described in this chapter, one being to focus on the consumer's purchasing power. From this approach has come the idea of using the mental health treatment system itself as a source of employment opportunities for its customers – either in treatment roles or in allied services – and the concept of the consumer-oriented pharmacy. We also looked at the viability of housing cooperatives as a way to advance the economic welfare and expand the productive roles of people with mental illness.

The second innovative approach we discussed is to focus on the individual consumer's business interests and to develop business incubators that help consumers to launch profitable small enterprises. Regardless of the successes or failures of these particular innovations, we have to recognise that innovation in general is essential if people with mental illness are to escape the poverty, idleness and social exclusion that have been their plight. What we have been doing so far has not been good enough.

Inclusion and empowerment of consumers

14.1 Consumer advocacy

Among the most important developments in psychiatry in the past 30 years, some would argue, has been the growth of organisations of relatives of people with serious mental illness. In the USA, the National Alliance for the Mentally Ill has lobbied for improvements in services for people with mental illness, for the direction of psychiatric resources towards those with the most severe disorders, and for increased research on schizophrenia. Media reports on mentally ill people have become less negative in response to a drive by the Alliance to establish a new openness and tolerance of psychiatric illness. In Britain, the National Schizophrenia Fellowship, now known as Rethink, established a few years earlier than its US counterpart, has been similarly active in providing support for its members, lobbying for needed services, fostering public education and sponsoring research. Its publications have covered such topics as inadequate services, mental health law and the importance of work for mentally disabled people. In Australia, SANE has mounted a strong country-wide anti-stigma campaign and is involved closely in the shaping of mental health policy.

There has also been growth in the organisation of primary consumers of mental health services in recent decades. The consumer, consumer/survivor or service-user movement, while gaining prominence in many parts of the world, is somewhat fragmented in comparison with the relatives' network. A listing of some of the important service-user organisations in Britain illustrates both the growing strength and the lack of cohesion of the movement – Mind, InterAction, the Hearing Voices Network, Survivors Speak Out, MadPride, Survivors' United Network, African Caribbean Users/Survivors Forum, MindLink, Manic Depression Fellowship, the Self Harm Network, the United Kingdom Advocacy Network, the Campaign Against Psychiatric Oppression, the National Voices Forum, the British Network for Alternatives to Psychiatry, and so on.

In the USA, there is a similar proliferation of consumer groups. Two prominent organisations, the National Mental Health Consumer Association and the National Alliance for Mental Patients, vie for membership, sponsor national conferences, send speakers to professional meetings, combat stigma through media presentations and lobby for political objectives. Recovery Inc. is a well-developed organisation with local chapters across the USA, and the National Empowerment Center is another prominent group. At the state level, there is often more organisational unity; California, Ohio and New York have particularly active consumer organisations.

Some groups, such as the National Mental Health Consumers Self-Help Clearinghouse, the National Empowerment Center, On Our Own and Schizophrenics Anonymous, focus primarily on providing support, information and advocacy for their members. Others are vigorously involved in advocating for human rights and in confronting the psychiatric profession on philosophical issues. The MindFreedom Support Coalition International launched a hunger strike in 2004 to draw attention to its campaign against biomedical hegemony in psychiatry and in support of its demand that the American Psychiatric Association (APA) produce evidence that schizophrenia is a real illness. The group's mission is to lead 'a nonviolent revolution of freedom, equality, truth and human rights that unites people affected by the mental health system with movements for justice everywhere' (www.mindfreedom.org). The organisation mounts demonstrations at major professional meetings against the practice of involuntary treatment and the use of restraints and seclusion in psychiatric units. It has criticised the extent to which the pharmaceutical industry influences policy and practice in psychiatry and at the time of writing is opposing a drug-company-sponsored proposal, supported by the Bush administration, to screen all US children for mental disorder. The group operates an Internet listserv called Dendron, which alerts over 2000 subscribers to issues of current importance. The organisation considers government support of consumer groups to be a form of co-optation that undermines their independence and their capacity for human rights activism.

Philosophical disagreements over such issues as involuntary treatment and whether mental illness really exists reinforce the tendency for splintering of consumer groups. Consumer leadership is also held back by the fact that many people who develop a psychotic disorder do so before they are old enough to have gained experience of how organisations work. The fragmentation of the primary consumer movement, however, has not prevented it from becoming involved in governance of the system of care and changing the face of mental health service delivery.

14.2 People with mental illness running their own treatment services

Consumers of mental health services have become increasingly involved in the governance of treatment services and in setting up their own services. In half of the states in the USA, consumers have been appointed to paid positions in the state mental health administrative offices. State regulations in California require that the boards of residential facilities include consumer members. Mental health agencies in Colorado are directed to hire a consumer manager to sit on the agency's executive committee. At the Mental Health Center of Boulder County in Colorado, people with serious mental illness are members of the governing board, various advisory boards, the board of the agency's fund-raising foundation and the quality-improvement committee. It has become the norm across the USA for consumers to be involved in service management at various levels, and, increasingly, they are developing their own services.

Consumer organisations have established drop-in centres, support groups, speakers' bureaus, telephone hotlines and a variety of other services. One consumer action group in Denver opened its own psychiatric clinic: the Capitol Hill Action and Recreation Group (CHARG) is a coalition of consumers and professionals that has established a consumer-run drop-in centre and a full-service psychiatric clinic for the treatment of people with serious mental illness. The clinic is accountable directly to an elected consumer board and to a second board comprised of professionals and other interested people. All matters of clinic policy require the consent of the consumer board. CHARG also provides consumer advocates for patients at the local state hospital, in boarding homes and in other locations.

Drop-in centre

We have a basement in the old post office and we're open five days a week for people with mental illness that have no place to go. The staff are all volunteers. We have a computer for those that would like to learn, and a quiet room for those that would like to be by themselves and listen to music and play games. We offer free coffee and pastries, companionship and different services. We offer classes and a group for people that want to talk about managing drugs and alcohol better. There's a fund for social activities. It's a place for people to come to share, when it's open.

Spiritmenders Community Center in inner-city San Francisco was established by the San Francisco Network of Mental Health Clients. The programme is run democratically and is funded and maintained solely by mental health service consumers. It offers a number of activities, a safe place to drop in and socialise (important in the inner city) and education for its members and the general public. It aims to empower its members through peer counselling and advocacy and by fostering self-advocacy. Members clearly do not see the centre as being part of the traditional mental health system. As one of the organisers frames their goal: 'Efforts are made to prevent those situations that force individuals to receive involuntary services and/or other mental health services.' Spiritmenders was one of the first of a now growing number of local consumer drop-in and support centres in the USA.

14.3 The psychosocial clubhouse model and its diffusion

Although consumer-run services are becoming more widespread, so too are collaborative provider/consumer models. Organisations such as Fountain House in New York City and Thresholds in Chicago have gained international prominence by establishing a model in which people with mental illness are involved in running a programme that meets many of their recreational, social and vocational needs. In these programmes, clients are referred to as 'members' and work with staff in running the operations of the clubhouse – putting together the daily newsletter, working in the food service or staffing the reception desk. The clubhouse is open in the evenings, at weekends and over holidays, providing a refuge for people who may live in cramped, cheerless housing and sometimes cannot fit in well in other social settings. Clubhouses are physically separated from the mental health treatment agency, and psychiatric treatment is definitively not part of the programme. The emphasis instead is on developing work skills and job opportunities for the members.

The clubhouse

I come in and answer the phones a couple times a week and I have a place to go when I've been in my apartment too long and I need to get out and see people. So I've been glad I've had the clubhouse. I can get a good meal if I don't feel like cooking. It keeps me focused during the week. I have some place to go and socialise and it's been a really nice experience.

A good example is the Chinook Clubhouse in Boulder, CO, which is modelled on Fountain House and operates a supported employment programme that locates jobs for the members in local businesses and trains and supports them as they settle into the new work. In preparation for this opportunity, members join clubhouse work groups like those at Fountain House. The programme is not for everyone: some lower-functioning clients may be scared off by the emphasis on work and many higher-functioning clients are not keen to mingle with other mentally ill people. A substantial number, nevertheless, take part in the programme and report a distinct improvement in their quality of life.

The story of the diffusion of the clubhouse model is of interest. Fountain House was founded in 1947 by ex-patients of Rockland State Hospital and for 30 years was the only one of its kind, enjoying an international reputation and entertaining hundreds of visitors each year. In 1976 Fountain House launched a national training programme and in 1988 a national expansion effort. The International Center for Clubhouse Development was established in 1994, along with a programme to certify clubhouses that met their standards of operation (Macias et al., 2001). By 2003, there were over 300 certified clubhouses worldwide, 191 in the USA, 29 in Scandinavia, 23 in Canada and 22 in Great Britain. In addition, Australia, New Zealand, Japan, Korea, Germany and Russia had established several such programmes (International Center for Clubhouse Development, 2004).

The clubhouse

I definitely would have to say the clubhouse has helped. It has given me a place to go. No matter what condition I'm in, I can come here. It's good to get out of the house. When I'm in really bad condition, I know I can come to the clubhouse. It's a help being around other people, seeing them in worse condition and better condition. They're pleasant and they're very supportive, and the clubhouse has even pushed me. It'll push me into jobs. I think that has helped me. I think the structure and being around other people and taking my mind off my problems have all helped me not focus on my illness.

A big thing for me was I learned computers at the clubhouse. I wouldn't have if I'd had to take a class. I know I would've gotten really frustrated and walked out. But learning computers at the clubhouse was so slow and easy, like, 'Oh, could you come over and help me with this?' 'Here's how you do this.' Now I've got my own computer and it was just such a big help for me to learn computers. The pace and ease of the clubhouse made it possible.

The clubhouse-certification process evaluates whether certain basic components of the clubhouse model are in place. Foremost among these is, what clubhouse organisers refer to as the 'work-ordered day' – a structured eight-hour day in which members and staff work side by side on clubhouse work units. New members are required to volunteer for work only when they feel ready; however, since they are assigned to a work group upon enrolment, the gentle pressure to become involved is always present. Another crucial element of the model is the democratic mode of decision-making and governance. Members and staff meet in open session to discuss policy and planning; no staff-only or member-only meetings are permitted. Other basic components that the certification team looks for include employment programmes, such as transitional employment; evening, weekend and holiday programmes; and community support and reach-out to members (Macias *et al.*, 2001; International Center for Clubhouse Development, 2004).

The attractions of the model for people with mental illness, most of whom are not well-off, include good cheap food, a comfortable social environment, a sense of community and mutual support, empowerment (which flows from the democratic philosophy) and access to employment. Researchers, however, point out weaknesses of the model. The clubhouse movement has conducted almost no randomised control trials and consequently has a weak evidence base. Clubhouse organisers, therefore, cannot specify which clubhouse elements are effective and which standards are necessary for success.

Given the strengths and potential weaknesses of this model and its delayed pattern of diffusion around the world, it is intriguing to reflect upon which factors have enhanced its adoption and which may yet present obstacles. Mandiberg (2000) suggests that it is important to distinguish between 'in-paradigm' and 'out-of-paradigm' modes of diffusion. In-paradigm diffusion, he argues, is rational and evidence-based and more readily gains access to established resources and legitimacy, but it is slower and more expensive. Assertive community treatment and supported employment fit this mode of diffusion. Out-of-paradigm diffusion takes the form of a social movement that offers some legitimacy but proceeds in a different way: those who adopt the model are more likely to do so as a result of a 'conversion' experience, similar to a religious conversion. Consequently, out-of-paradigm diffusion is faster and more independent of the usual professional processes. The diffusion of the clubhouse model and, many would argue, early intervention in psychosis, appears to have taken this road.

There is, for example, a cult-like quality to the clubhouse movement. At international clubhouse meetings, adherents carry banners and chant 'Clubhouse! Clubhouse! Clubhouse!' For some people in the field, this is an obstacle to adoption. Another deterrent is the rigidity of the certification guidelines, which do not take into account cultural variations around family, gender politics, and so on (Mandiberg, 2000). Consequently, it is hard to predict the extent to which the global clubhouse network will expand in the future, although, to this point, its expansion has been vigorous.

It is intriguing to note that in the 1940s, when Fountain House was being established in New York City as an empowering community model for people with mental illness, another model that was based on power-sharing between staff and patients, the therapeutic community, was being introduced into British hospitals. The therapeutic community, along with other changes in hospital management, was effective in helping long-hospitalised patients shake off the effects of the institutional neurosis – the passive withdrawal, posturing, restless pacing and sudden aggressiveness that was a product of the years of restrictions, regimentation and emptiness of hospital confinement. The therapeutic community served its purpose, allowing many patients to move to the community as they regained their functional skills; since then, however, it has mostly faded away. The same active ingredient in the clubhouse model – transferring power from the treatment providers to the person with mental illness – continues to serve a valuable purpose to this day in combating what we might term the 'existential neurosis' – the alienation, meaninglessness and boredom that afflicts many people with serious mental illness living in the community.

14.4 The recovery model

Recognition of the importance of combating alienation and empowering consumers and of the potential for good outcome in serious mental illness has gained the force of a social movement. This vision, which has come to be termed the 'recovery model', is influencing service development in the USA, Britain and many other countries. The model refers both to the subjective experiences of hope, healing, empowerment and interpersonal support experienced by people with mental illness, their carers and service providers, and to the creation of recovery-oriented services that engender a positive culture of healing and a support for human rights. Flowing from this model is a renewed interest in many of the concepts that we have dwelt upon in this book, including:

- fighting the stigma that leads people with mental illness to lose their sense of self;
- providing access to services and education that give consumers the knowledge and skills to manage their illnesses;
- empowering consumers to share responsibility with providers in the healing process;
- providing access to peer support that validates the possibility of recovery.

The model calls for professionals to provide services in which decisions about treatment are taken collaboratively with the consumer, and for the creation of consumer-run services that offer advocacy, mentoring and peer support via such mechanisms as consumer-run 'warm-lines' (peer-to-peer supportive chatlines) and drop-in centres. Collaborative models, such as the psychosocial clubhouse and educational programmes that involve both professionals and consumers as teachers, are seen as important elements of recovery-oriented services (Jacobson and Greenley, 2001).

Optimism about recovery

Something that contributed to my recovery was seeing that movie called *A Beautiful Mind*. This great mathematician, John whatever-his-name was, at Princeton. He also suffered from this illness, and I could identify with exactly what was going on in the movie. And he, after how many years, I don't know, he wasn't on medication. But he could spot when the illness surfaced and he knew not to pay any attention to it. That was a great inspiration to me because I didn't know that that stage could be reached. That is something that I hope to attain myself.

The recovery process

If I get, like, crying, mad, with the voices arguing in my head, I say, 'It's a time problem.' I'm getting better with time, and I got some getting better to do. I understand that it is schizophrenia and you can grow out of it. I'm just convinced I'm going to. And I keep telling myself, 'It's a time problem.' I may not be able to work out the problem right now, but in time I'll be able to solve this problem.

I guess it has helped me to separate what is the illness and what is me. I really have a belief that I'm going to grow out of my illness, these voices in my head. I mean, I'll still have the simple discussion of which dress to wear today, but the arguments and the negativity my voices push on me, that's all going to disappear. And, it's nice to know that that's going to go away. It gives me some hope.

The roots of the recovery model may be found in both the consumer/survivor movement and professional psychiatric rehabilitation initiatives. Consumer activists have reinforced the drive towards empowerment, collaboration and recognition of human rights. Rehabilitation professionals, on the other hand, have emphasised the need for best practices in treatment that recognise the value of work and a sense of community in the lives of people with mental illness and the importance of environmental factors in helping people with psychiatric disorders achieve their best functioning potential (Jacobson and Curtis, 2000). Many practitioners have emphasised that, far from there being a conflict between evidence-based treatment practices and the recovery model, a marriage between these two areas of interest provides an opportunity for achieving optimal outcomes (Torrey *et al.*, 2005). Some observers argue that the marriage between these two approaches will be stronger if consumers are involved in conducting research and in planning and implementing evidence-based programmes. In line with this recommendation, a joint user/professional research planning group has been established at the Institute of Psychiatry in London. Observers also suggest that professional schools should recruit more consumers into their training programmes, and that professionals who have experienced mental illness themselves should feel free to speak out about the experience of illness and the benefits of evidence-based practice (Freese *et al.*, 2001).

The recovery process

Age has a lot to do with recovery. Growing more patient. Having experience and the ability to sift through what was and what is. Being open to failure or success. I'm pretty new in recovery and pretty enthusiastic, but I'm learning from the people ahead of me.

14.5 Conclusions

We have every reason to be positive about the future for people with mental illness. In the past decade, we have seen many community organisations, professional groups, governmental bodies and commercial entities join the columns fighting the stigma of mental illness, laying siege to one of the last bastions of prejudice and discrimination to be found in the more enlightened societies. A dramatic increase in awareness of this type is an essential first step in changing attitudes and behaviour towards any marginalised group. More professionals and policymakers are recognising that the social exclusion of people with mental illness breeds a form of self-stigmatisation among those with mental illness that impedes recovery. We have developed more effective methods for minimising symptoms of psychosis, for enhancing functioning and for aiding integration into the community. We now know that work helps people recover from serious mental illness. Better still, we have developed effective ways for getting people with mental illness back to work. We understand, moreover, that consumer involvement and empowerment are of crucial importance in promoting recovery from mental illness, and we are making steps to ensure that these elements are built into our treatment and rehabilitation programmes.

> **Empowerment**
>
> I was able to self-monitor my medication. That made me feel pretty empowered. It made me feel as if I could use my own mind to seek sanity. If I could keep track of whether I needed to take medication or not, which sometimes didn't happen, seemed to lead to the idea that I could make some sort of progress in other areas. Including figuring out why in the heck I went to see the doctor in the first place.

One more thing has become clear. The task of integrating people with mental illness into society is not just the business of mental health professionals. It is a task that demands a partnership between these same professionals, people with mental illness themselves, family members and many others. It involves communications specialists and employers, police officers and teachers, businesspeople and landlords, advocates and lawyers, children and politicians – it involves all of us.

References

Ahr, P. R., Gorodezky, M. J. and Cho, D. W. (1981). Measuring the relationship of public psychiatric admissions to rising unemployment. *Hospital and Community Psychiatry*, **32**, 398–401.

American Psychiatric Association (1994). *Diagnostic and Statistical Manual of Mental Disorders*, 4th edn. Washington, DC: American Psychiatric Press.

Anderson, C. M., Hogarty, G., Bayer, T. and Needleman, R. (1984). Expressed emotion and social networks of parents of schizophrenic patients. *British Journal of Psychiatry*, **144**, 247–55.

Anderson, J., Dayson, D., Wills, W., *et al.* (1993). The TAPS project 13: clinical and social outcomes of long-stay psychiatric patients after one year in the community. *British Journal of Psychiatry*, **162** (Suppl. 19), 45–56.

Andrews, B. and Brown, G. W. (1991). *The Self Evaluation and Social Support (SESS) Manual*. London: Royal Holloway and Bedford New College.

Angell, B. and Test, M. A. (2002). The relationship of clinical factors and environmental opportunities to social functioning in young adults with schizophrenia. *Schizophrenia Bulletin*, **28**, 259–71.

Angermeyer, M. C. (2000). Schizophrenia and violence. *Acta Psychiatrica Scandinavica*, **102** (Suppl. 407), 63–7.

Angermeyer, M. C. and Matschinger, H. (1996). The effect of personal experience with mental illness on the attitude towards individuals suffering from mental disorders. *Social Psychiatry and Psychiatric Epidemiology*, **31**, 321–6.

Angermeyer, M. C. and Matschinger, H. (1997). Social representations of mental illness among the public. In *The Image of Madness*, ed. J. Guimon, W. Fischer and N. Sartorius. Basel: Karger, pp. 20–28.

Anthony, W. A., Buell, G. W., Sharatt, S. and Althoff, M. D. (1972). The efficacy of psychiatric rehabilitation. *Psychological Bulletin*, **78**, 447–56.

Anthony, W. A., Cohen, M. R. and Danley, K. S. (1988). The psychiatric rehabilitation model as applied to vocational rehabilitation. In *Vocational Rehabilitation of Persons with Prolonged Psychiatric Disorders*, ed. J. A. Cardiello and M. D. Bell. Baltimore, MD: Johns Hopkins University Press, pp. 59–80.

Anthony, W. A., Rogers, E. S., Cohen, M. and Davis, R. R. (1995). Relationship between psychiatric symptomatology, work skills, and future vocational performance. *Psychiatric Services*, **46**, 353–8.

Arboleda-Flórez, J. (1998). Mental illness and violence: an epidemiological appraisal of the evidence. *Canadian Journal of Psychiatry*, **43**, 989–96.

Astrachan, B. M., Brauer, L., Harrow, M., *et al.* (1974). Symptomatic outcome in schizophrenia. *Archives of General Psychiatry*, **31**, 155–60.

Averett, S., Warner, R., Little, J. and Huxley, P. (1999). Labor supply, disability benefits and mental illness. *Eastern Economic Journal*, **25**, 279–88.

Bachrach, L. L. (1976). *Deinstitutionalization: An Analytic Review and Sociological Perspective.* Rockville, MD: National Institute of Mental Health.

Bailey, E. L., Ricketts, S. K., Becker, D. R., *et al.* (1998). Do long-term day treatment clients benefit from supported employment? *Psychiatric Rehabilitation Journal*, **22**, 24–9.

Ball, R. A., Moore, E. and Kuipers, E. (1992). Expressed emotion in community care staff: a comparison of patient outcome in a nine month follow-up of two hostels. *Social Psychiatry and Psychiatric Epidemiology*, **27**, 35–9.

Barham, P. and Hayward, R. (1996). The lives of 'users'. In *Mental Health Matters: A Reader*, ed. T. Heller, J. Reynolds, R. Gomm, R. Muston and S. Pattison. London: Macmillan, p. 232.

Barnes, J. and Thornicroft, G. (1993). The last resort? Bed and breakfast accommodation for mentally ill people in a seaside town. *Health Trends*, **25**, 87–90.

Barrowclough, C., Tarrier, N., Humphreys, L., Ward, J. and Gregg L. (2003). Self-esteem in schizophrenia: relationship between self-evaluation, family attitudes and symptomatology. *Journal of Abnormal Psychology*, **112**, 92–9.

Barton, R. (1976). *Institutional Neurosis*, 3rd edn. Bristol: J. Wright.

Bassuk, E. L. (1984). The homeless problem. *Scientific American*, **6**, 40–45.

Beck, A. T. (1976). *Cognitive Therapy and the Emotional Disorders.* New York: International University Press.

Becker, D. R. and Bond, G. R. (2002). *Supported Employment Implementation Resource Kit.* Rockville, MD: Center for Mental Health Services, Substance Abuse and Mental Health Services Administration.

Becker, D. R. and Drake, R. E. (2003). *A Working Life for People with Severe Mental Illness.* New York: Oxford University Press.

Becker, D. R., Bebout, R. R. and Drake, R. E. (1998). Job preferences of people with severe mental illness: a replication. *Psychiatric Rehabilitation Journal*, **22**, 46–50.

Becker, D. R., Bond, G. R., McCarthy, D., *et al.* (2001). Converting day treatment centers to supported employment programs in Rhode Island. *Psychiatric Services*, **52**, 351–7.

Bedell, J. R., Draving, D., Parrish, A., *et al.* (1998). A description and comparison of experiences of people with mental disorders in supported employment and paid prevocational training. *Psychiatric Rehabilitation Journal*, **21**, 279–83.

Bell, M. D. and Lysaker, P. H. (1997). Clinical benefits of paid work activity in schizophrenia: 1-year followup. *Schizophrenia Bulletin*, **23**, 317–28.

Bell, M. D., Milstein, R. M. and Lysaker, P. H. (1993). Pay as an incentive in work participation by patients with severe mental illness. *Hospital and Community Psychiatry*, **44**, 684–6.

Bell, M. D., Lysaker, P. H. and Milstein, R.M. (1996). Clinical benefits of paid work activity in schizophrenia. *Schizophrenia Bulletin*, **22**, 51–67.

Bennett, R. (1995). The Crisis Home Program of Dane County. In *Alternatives to Hospital for Acute Psychiatric Treatment*, ed. R. Warner. Washington, DC: American Psychiatric Press, pp. 227–36.

Berkowitz, M. and Hill, M. A. (1986). *Disability and the Labor Market: Economic Problems, Policies, and Programs*. Ithaca, NY: ILR Press.

Black, B. J. (1992). A kind word for sheltered work. *Psychosocial Rehabilitation Journal*, **15**, 87–9.

Bleuler, M. (1978). *The Schizophrenic Disorders: Long-Term Patient and Family Studies* (trans. S. M. Clemens). New Haven and London: Yale University Press.

Bond, G. R. (1984). An economic analysis of psychosocial rehabilitation. *Hospital and Community Psychiatry*, **35**, 356–62.

Bond, G. R. (1992). Vocational rehabilitation. In *Handbook of Psychiatric Rehabilitation*, ed. R. P. Liberman. New York: Macmillan Press, pp 244–63.

Bond, G. R. (1998). Principles of individual placement and support. *Psychiatric Rehabilitation Journal*, **22**, 11–23.

Bond, G. R. (2001). Implementing supported employment as an evidence-based practice. *Psychiatric Services*, **52**, 313–22.

Bond G. R. (2004a). Supported employment: an evidence-based practice. Presented at Ohio SAMI CCOE Conference, Columbus, OH, 27 September.

Bond, G. R. (2004b). Supported employment: evidence for an evidence-based practice. *Psychiatric Rehabilitation Journal*, **27**, 345–59.

Bond, G. R., Dietzen, L. L., McGrew, J. H. and Miller, L. D. (1995). Accelerating entry into supported employment for persons with severe psychiatric disabilities. *Rehabilitation Psychology*, **40**, 91–111.

Bond, G. R., Resnick, S. R., Drake, R. E., *et al.* (2001). Does competitive employment improve nonvocational outcomes for people with severe mental illness? *Journal of Consulting and Clinical Psychology*, **65**, 489–501.

Boydall, K. M., Trainor, J. M. and Pierri, A. M. (1989). The effect of group homes for the mentally ill on residential property values. *Hospital and Community Psychiatry*, **40**, 957–8.

Boyles, P. (1988). Mentally ill gain a foothold in working world. *Boston Sunday Globe*, 5 June.

Bradshaw, J., Hicks, L. and Parker, H. (1992). Summary Budget Standards for Six Households. Working paper 12. Family Budget Unit York, Department of Social Policy, University of York, York.

Brekke, J. S., Levin, S., Wolkon, G. H., *et al.* (1993). Psychosocial functioning and subjective experience in schizophrenia. *Schizophrenia Bulletin*, **19**, 599–608.

Brekke, J. S., Ansell, M., Long, J., *et al.* (1999). Intensity and continuity of services and functional outcomes in the rehabilitation of persons with schizophrenia. *Psychiatric Services*, **50**, 248–56.

Brenner, M. H. (1973). *Mental Illness and the Economy*. Cambridge, MA: Harvard University Press.

Brockington, I. F., Hall, P. H., Levings, J., *et al.* (1993). The community's tolerance of the mentally ill. *British Journal of Psychiatry*, **162**, 93–9.

Bromley, J. S. and Cunningham, S. J. (2004). 'You don't bring me flowers any more': an investigation into the experience of stigma by psychiatric in-patients. *Psychiatric Bulletin*, **28**, 371–4.

Brown, P. (1985). *The Transfer of Care: Psychiatric Deinstitutionalisation and its Aftermath*. Henley-on-Thames: Routledge.

Brown, G. W. and Rutter, M. (1966). The measurement of family activities and relationships: a methodological study. *Human Relations*, **19**, 241–63.

Brown, G. W., Carstairs, G. M. and Topping, G. (1958). Post-hospital adjustment of chronic mental patients. *Lancet*, **ii**, 685–9.

Bryson, G., Lysaker, P. and Bell, M. (2002). Quality of life benefits of paid work activity in schizophrenia. *Schizophrenia Bulletin*, **28**, 249–57.

Budson, R. (1983). Residential care for the chronic mentally ill. In *The Chronic Psychiatric Patient in the Community: Principles of Treatment*, ed. I. Barofsky and R. D. Budson. New York: SP Medical and Scientific Books, pp. 285–6.

Butzlaff, R. L. and Hooley, J. M. (1999). Expressed emotion and psychiatric relapse: a meta-analysis. *Archives of General Psychiatry*, **55**, 547–52.

Carey, T. G., Owens, J. M. and Horne, P. (1993). An analysis of a new longstay population: the need for mental hospitals. *Irish Journal of Psychological Medicine*, **10**, 80–85.

Carrier, J. and Kendall, I. (1997). Evolution of policy. In *Care in the Community: Illusion or Reality?*, ed. J. Leff. Chichester: John Wiley & Sons, pp. 3–20.

Casper, E. S. and Fishbein, S. (2002). Job satisfaction and job success as moderators of the self-esteem of people with mental illness. *Rehabilitation Counseling Bulletin*, **26**, 33–42.

Caton, C. L. M., Shrout, P. E., Eagle, P. F., *et al.* (1994). Risk factors for homelessness among schizophrenic men: a case–control study. *American Journal of Public Health*, **84**, 265–70.

Chandler, D., Meisel, J., Hu, T.-W., *et al.* (1997). A capitated model for a cross-section of severely mentally ill clients: employment outcomes. *Community Mental Health Journal*, **33**, 501–16.

Chandler, D., Levin, S. and Barry, P. (1999). The menu approach to employment services: philosophy and five-year outcomes. *Psychiatric Rehabilitation Journal*, **23**, 24–33.

Cheetham, W. S. and Cheetham, R. J. (1976). Concepts of mental illness amongst the Xhosa people in South Africa. *Australian and New Zealand Journal of Psychiatry*, **10**, 39–45.

Ciompi, L. (1980). Catamnestic long-term study on the course of life and ageing of schizophrenics. *Schizophrenia Bulletin*, **5**, 606–18.

Clausen, J. A. (1981). Stigma and mental disorder: phenomena and terminology. *Psychiatry*, **44**, 287–96.

Consumer Health Sciences (1997). *The Schizophrenia Patient Project: Brief Summary of Results – September 1997*. Princeton, NJ: Consumer Health Sciences.

Cooper, B. (1961). Social class and prognosis in schizophrenia: parts I and II. *Journal of Preventive and Social Medicine*, **15**, 17–30, 31–41.

Creed, F., Black, D., Anthony, F., *et al.* (1990). Randomised controlled trial of day patient versus inpatient psychiatric treatment. *British Medical Journal*, **300**, 1033–7.

Crisp, A. H., Gelder, M. G., Rix, S., Meltzer, H. I. and Rowlands, O. J. (2000). Stigmatization of people with mental illnesses. *British Journal of Psychiatry*, **177**, 4–7.

Cumming, E. and Cumming, J. (1957). *Closed Ranks: An Experiment in Mental Health Education*. Cambridge, MA: Harvard University Press.

Davis, A. and Betteridge, J. (1997). Welfare to Work: Benefit Issues for People with Mental Health Problems. Briefing No. 10. London: Mental Health Foundation.

Davis, M. and Thompson, B. (1992). *Cooperative Housing: A Development Primer*. Washington, DC: National Cooperative Business Association.

Davis, J. M., Chen, N. and Glick, I. D. (2003). A meta-analysis of the efficacy of 2nd-generation antipsychotics. *Archives of General Psychiatry*, **60**, 553–64.

Dayson, D. (1992). The TAPS project 15: the social networks of two group homes: a pilot study. *Journal of Mental Health*, **1**, 99–106.

Dear, M., Clark, G. and Clark, S. (1979). Economic cycles and mental health care policy: an examination of the macro-context for social service planning. *Social Science and Medicine*. **136**, 43–53.

Delaney, K. R. and Fogg, L. (2005). Patient characteristics and setting variables related to the use of restraint on four inpatient psychiatric units for youths. *Psychiatric Services*, **56**, 186–92.

Dell'Acqua, G. and Dezza, M. G. C. (1985). The end of the mental hospital: a review of the psychiatric experience in Trieste. *Acta Psychiatrica Scandinavica Supplementum* **316**, 45–69.

Dick, N. and Shepherd, G. (1994). Work and mental health: a preliminary test of Warr's model in sheltered workshops for the mentally ill. *Journal of Mental Health*, **3**, 387–400.

Dilk, M. N. and Bond, G. R. (1996). Meta-analytic evaluation of skills training research for individuals with severe mental illness. *Journal of Consulting and Clinical Psychology*, **64**, 1337–46.

Disability Income Group (1997). *Investing in Disabled People: A Strategy from Welfare to Work*. London: Disability Income Group.

Doherty, E. G. (1976). Labeling effects in psychiatric hospitalisation: a study of diverging patterns in inpatient self-labeling processes. *Archives of General Psychiatry*. **32**, 562–8.

Donat, D. C. (2003). An analysis of successful efforts to reduce the use of seclusion and restraint at a public psychiatric hospital. *Psychiatric Services*, **54**, 1119–23.

Donnelly, M. (1992). *The Politics of Mental Health in Italy*. London: Routledge.

Drake, R. E., Becker, D. R., Biesanz, J. C., *et al.* (1994). Rehabilitation day treatment vs. supported employment: 1. Vocational outcomes. *Community Mental Health Journal*, **30**, 519–32.

Drake, R. E., Becker, D. R., Biesanz, J. C. (1996). Day treatment versus supported employment for persons with severe mental illness: a replication study. *Psychiatric Services*, **47**, 1125–7.

Drake, R. E., Becker, D. R., Bond, G. R. and Mueser, K. T. (2003). A process analysis of integrated and non-integrated approaches to supported employment. *Journal of Vocational Rehabilitation*, **18**, 51–8.

Drew, D., Drebing, C. E., Van Ormer, A., *et al.* (2001). Effects of disability compensation on participation in and outcomes of vocational rehabilitation. *Psychiatric Services*, **52**, 1479–84.

Drury, V., Birchwood, M., Cochrane, R., *et al.* (1996). Cognitive therapy and recovery from acute psychosis: a controlled trial. 1. Impact on psychotic symptoms. *British Journal of Psychiatry*, **169**, 593–601.

Dunn, M., O'Driscoll, C., Dayson, D., Wills, W. and Leff, J. (1990). The TAPS project 4: an observational study of the social life of long-stay patients. *British Journal of Psychiatry*, **157**, 842–8.

Eisenberg, P. and Lazarsfeld, P. F. (1938). The psychological effects of unemployment. *Psychological Bulletin*, **35**, 358–90.

Ellwood, D. (1988). *Poor Support*. New York: Basic Books.

El-Islam, M. F. (1982). Rehabilitation of schizophrenics by the extended family. *Acta Psychiatrica Scandinavica*, **65**, 112–19.

Fioritti, A. (2004). Disincentives to work within the Italian disability pension system. Presented at the WPA International Congress on Treatments in Psychiatry: An Update, 10–13 November, Florence, Italy.

Fischer, E. P., Shumway, M. and Owen, R. R. (2002). Priorities of consumers, providers, and family members in the treatment of schizophrenia. *Psychiatric Services*, **53**, 724–9.

Fowler, D., Garety, P. A. and Kuipers, L. (1995). *Cognitive Behaviour Therapy for Psychosis: Theory and Practice*. Chichester: John Wiley & Sons.

Freeman, D. and Garety, P. A. (2004). *Paranoia: The Psychology of Persecutory Delusions*. Maudsley Monographs 45. Hove: Psychology Press.

Freeman, H. E. and Simmons, O. G. (1963). *The Mental Patient Comes Home*. New York: John Wiley & Sons.

Freeman, D., Garety, P. A., Bebbington, P., *et al.* (2005). Psychological investigation of the structure of paranoia in a non-clinical population. *British Journal of Psychiatry*, **186**, 427–35.

Freese, F. J., Stanley, J., Kress, K. and Vogel-Scibilia, S. (2001). Integrating evidence-based practices and the recovery model. *Psychiatric Services*, **52**, 1462–8.

Freud, S. (1930). Civilization and its discontents. In *Standard Edition of the Complete Psychological Works of Sigmund Freud*, ed. J. Strachey, vol. 21. London: Hogarth Press.

Fromkin, K. R. (1985). Gender differences among chronic schizophrenics in the perceived helpfulness of community-based treatment programs. Unpublished Ph. D. thesis. Department of Psychology, University of Colorado, Boulder, CO.

Gallo, K. M. (1994). First person account: self-stigmatization. *Schizophrenia Bulletin*, **20**, 407–10.

Gatherer, A. and Reid, J. J. A. (1963). *Public Attitudes and Mental Health Education*. Northampton: Northamptonshire Health Department.

Giel, R., Gezaghen, Y. and van Luijk, J. N. (1968). Faith-healing and spirit-possession in Ghion, Ethiopia. *Social Science and Medicine*, **2**, 63–79.

Goffman, E. (1963). *Stigma: Notes on the Management of Spoiled Identity*. Englewood Cliffs, NJ: Prentice-Hall.

Gold, M. and Marrone, J. (1998). Mass Bay Employment Services (a service of Bay Cove Human Services, Inc.): a story of leadership, vision, and action resulting in employment for people with mental illness. *Roses and Thorns from the Grassroots*, **spring**.

Gowdy, E. A., Carlson, L. S. and Rapp, C. A. (2003). Practices differentiating high-performing from low-performing supported employment programs. *Psychiatric Rehabilitation Journal*, **26**, 232–9.

Greden, J. F. and Tandon, R. (1995). Long-term treatment for lifetime disorders? *Archives of General Psychiatry*, **52**, 197–200.

Grove, R. (2004). Disincentives to work in the UK welfare system – and how to overcome them. Presented at the WPA International Congress on Treatments in Psychiatry: An Update, 10–13 November Florence, Italy.

Grove, B., Freudenberg, M., Harding, A. and O'Flynn, D. (1997). *The Social Firm Handbook*. Brighton: Pavilion Publishing.

Guinness, E. A. (1992). Patterns of mental illness in the early stages of urbanisation. *British Journal of Psychiatry*, **160** (Suppl. 16), 24–41.

Gunderson, J. G. and Mosher, L. R. (1975). The cost of schizophrenia. *American Journal of Psychiatry*, **132**, 901–6.

Hall, P. L. and Tarrier, N. (2003). The cognitive-behavioural treatment of low self-esteem in psychotic patients: a pilot study. *Behaviour Research and Therapy*, **41**, 317–32.

Harding, E. (2005). Partners in care: service user employment in the NHS – a user's perspective. *Psychiatric Bulletin*, **29**, 268–9.

Harding, C. M., Brooks, G. W., Ashikaga, T., *et al.* (1987). The Vermont longitudinal study of persons with severe mental illness. I. Methodology, study samples, and overall status 32 years later. *American Journal of Psychiatry*, **144**, 718–26.

Harrison, G., Hopper, K., Craig, T., *et al.* (2001). Recovery from psychotic illness: a 15- and 25-year international follow-up study. *British Journal of Psychiatry*, **178**, 506–17.

Hart, A. F. (1982). Policy responses to schizophrenia: support for the vulnerable family. *Home Health Services Quarterly*, **3**, 225–41.

Hartl, K. (1992). A-Way Express: a way to empowerment through employment. *Canadian Journal of Community Mental Health*, **11**, 73–7.

Herzberg, J. (1987). No fixed abode: a comparison of men and women admitted to an East London psychiatric hospital. *British Journal of Psychiatry*, **150**, 621–7.

Hollingshead, A. B. and Redlich, F. C. (1958). *Social Class and Mental Illness*. New York: John Wiley & Sons.

Holzner, B., Kemmler, G. and Meise, U. (1998). The impact of work-related rehabilitation on the quality of life of patients with schizophrenia. *Social Psychiatry and Psychiatric Epidemiology*, **33**, 624–31.

Huber, G., Gross, G. and Schuttler, R. (1975). A long-term follow-up study of schizophrenia: psychiatric course of illness and prognosis. *Acta Psychiatrica Scandinavica*, **52**, 49–75.

International Center for Clubhouse Development (2004). *International Clubhouse Directory 2003*. New York: International Center for Clubhouse Development.

Jablensky, A., Sartorius, N., Ernberg, G., *et al.* (1992). Schizophrenia: manifestations, incidence and course in different cultures. A World Health Organization ten-country study. *Psychological Medicine Monograph Supplement*, **20**, 97.

Jacobson, N. and Curtis, L. (2000). Recovery as policy in mental health services: strategies emerging from the states. *Psychiatric Rehabilitation Journal*, **23**, 333–41.

Jacobson, N. and Greenley, D. (2001). What is recovery? A conceptual model and explication. *Psychiatric Services*, **52**, 482–5.

Johns, L. C., Cannon, M., Singleton, N., *et al.* (2004). Prevalence and correlates of self-reported symptoms in the British population. *British Journal of Psychiatry*, **185**, 298–305.

Jones, D. (1993). The TAPS project. 11: the selection of patients for reprovision. *British Journal of Psychiatry*, **162** (Suppl. 19), 36–9.

Jorm, A. F., Korten, A. E., Jacomb, P. A., *et al.* (1997). 'Mental health literacy': a survey of the public's ability to recognise mental disorders and their beliefs about the effectiveness of treatment. *Medical Journal of Australia*, **166**, 182–6.

Jorm, A. F., Korten, A. E. and Jacomb, P. A. (1999). Attitudes towards people with a mental disorder: a survey of the Australian public and health professionals. *Australian and New Zealand Journal of Psychiatry*, **33**, 77–83.

Kakutani, K. (1998). New Life Espresso: report on a business run by people with psychiatric disabilities. *Psychiatric Rehabilitation Journal*, **22**, 111–15.

Kapur, S. and Seeman, P. (2001). Does fast dissociation from the dopamine D_2 receptor explain the action of atypical antipsychotics? A new hypothesis. *American Journal of Psychiatry*, **158**, 360–69.

Karidi, M. J., Tzedaki, M., Papakonstantinou, K., *et al.* (2006). Preliminary results of an ongoing study, administering the Self-Stigmatising Questionnaire to schizophrenic outpatients. *World Psychiatry*, in press.

Kates, N., Nikolaou, L., Baillie, B. and Hess, J. (1997). An in-home employment program for people with mental illness. *Psychiatric Rehabilitation Journal*, **20**, 56–60.

Kaus, M. (1986). The work ethic state. *New Republic*, **7 July**, 22–33.

Kennard, D. and Clemmey, R. (1976). Psychiatric patients as seen by self and others: an exploration of change in a therapeutic community setting. *British Journal of Medical Psychology*, **49**, 35–53.

Killaspy, H., Dalton, J., McNicholas, S. and Johnson, S. (2000). Drayton Park, an alternative to hospital admission for women in acute mental health crisis. *Psychiatric Bulletin*, **24**, 101–4.

Killaspy, H., Harden, C., Holloway, F. and King, M. (2006). What do mental health rehabilitation services do and what are they for? *Journal of Mental Health*, **14**, 157–65.

Kingdon, D., Sharma, T., Hart, D. and the Schizophrenia Subgroup of the Royal College of Psychiatrists' Changing Minds Campaign (2004). What attitudes do psychiatrists hold towards people with mental illness? *Psychiatric Bulletin*, **28**, 401–6.

Kingham, M. and Corfe, M. (2005). Experiences of a mixed court liaison and diversion scheme. *Psychiatric Bulletin*, **29**, 137–40.

Kovess, V. (2002). The homeless mentally ill. In *Psychiatry in Society*, ed. N. Sartorius, W. Gaebel, J. J. López-Ibor and M. Maj. Chichester: John Wiley & Sons.

Kraepelin, E. (1896). *Dementia praecox*, 15th edn. Leipzig: Psychiatric Barth.

Krupa, T. (1998). The consumer-run business: people with psychiatric disabilities as entrepreneurs. *Work*, **11**, 3–10.

Kuipers, E., Garety, P., Fowler, D., *et al.* (1997). London–East Anglia randomised controlled trial of cognitive-behavioural therapy for psychosis. I: effects of the treatment phase. *British Journal of Psychiatry*, **171**, 319–27.

Kuipers, E., Fowler, D., Garety, P., *et al.* (1998). London–East Anglia randomised controlled trial of cognitive-behavioural therapy for psychosis. III: follow-up and economic evaluation at 18 months. *British Journal of Psychiatry*, **173**, 61–8.

Kuipers, E., Leff, J. and Lam, D. (2002). *Family Work for Schizophrenia: A Practical Guide*, 2nd edn. London: Gaskell.

Lamb, H. R. (1979). The new asylums in the community. *Archives of General Psychiatry*, **36**, 129–34.

Lamb, H. R. (1983). Serving long-term patients in the cities. In *The Chronic Psychiatric Patient in the Community: Principles of Treatment*, ed. I. Barofsky and R. D. Budson. New York: SP Medical and Scientific Books, pp. 411–12.

Lecomte, T., Cyr, M., Lesage, A. D., *et al.* (1999). *Journal of Nervous and Mental Diseases*, **187**, 406–13.

Lecomte, T., Wilde, J. B. and Wallace, C. J. (1999). Mental health consumers as peer interviewers. *Psychiatric Services*, **50**, 693–5.

Leff, J. (1988). *Psychiatry Around the Globe: A Transcultural View*. London: Gaskell.

Leff, J. (1997). The downside of reprovision. In *Care in the Community: Illusion or Reality?*, ed. J. Leff. Chichester: John Wiley & Sons.

Leff, J. (1998). MORI survey on public attitudes to schizophrenia. *Primary Care Psychiatry*, **4**, 107.

Leff, J. and Szmidla, A. (2002). Evaluation of a special rehabilitation programme for patients who are difficult to place. *Social Psychiatry and Psychiatric Epidemiology*, **37**, 1–5.

Leff, J. and Trieman, N. (2000). The TAPS project 46: long-stay patients discharged from psychiatric hospitals: social and clinical outcomes after five years in the community. *British Journal of Psychiatry*, **176**, 217–23.

Leff, J. and Vaughn, C. (1985). *Expressed Emotion in Families: Its Significance for Mental Illness*. New York: Guilford.

Leff, J., Kuipers, L., Berkowitz, R., Eberlein-Fries, R. and Sturgeon, D. (1982). A controlled trial of social intervention in the families of schizophrenic patients. *British Journal of Psychiatry*, **141**, 121–34.

Leff, J. Wig, N. N., Ghosh, A., *et al.* (1987). Expressed emotion and schizophrenia in North India. III. Influence of relatives' expressed emotion on the course of schizophrenia in Chandigarh. *British Journal of Psychiatry*, **151**, 166–73.

Leff, J., Tress, K. and Edwards, B. (1988). The clinical course of depressive symptoms in schizophrenia. *Schizophrenia Research*, **1**, 25–30.

Leff, J., O'Driscoll, C., Dayson, D., Wills, W. and Anderson, J. (1990). The TAPS project 5: the structure of social-network data obtained from long-stay patients. *British Journal of Psychiatry*, **157**, 848–52.

Leff, J., Thornicroft, G., Coxhead, N. and Crawford, C. (1994). The TAPS project 22: a five-year follow-up of long-stay psychiatric patients discharged to the community. *British Journal of Psychiatry*, **165** (Suppl. 25), 13–17.

Lefley, H. P. (1987). Impact of mental illness in families of mental health professionals. *Journal of Nervous and Mental Disease*, **175**, 277–85.

Lehman, A. F. (1988). A quality of life interview for the chronically mentally ill. *Evaluation and Program Planning*, **11**, 51–62.

Lehman, A. F. (1995). Vocational rehabilitation in schizophrenia. *Schizophrenia Bulletin*, **21**, 645–56.

Lehman, A. F. and Steinwachs, D. M. (1998). Patterns of usual care for schizophrenia: initial results from the Schizophrenia Patient Outcomes Research Team (PORT). client survey. *Schizophrenia Bulletin*, **24**, 11–20.

Liebow, E. (1967). *Talley's Corner: A Study of Negro Streetcorner Men*. Boston, MA: Little, Brown.

Link, B. and Cullen, F. T. (1986). Contact with the mentally ill and perceptions of how dangerous they are. *Journal of Health and Social Behavior*, **27**, 289–303.

Link, B. and Phelan, J. (2004). Fear of people with mental illness: the role of personal and impersonal contact and exposure to threat or harm. *Journal of Health and Social Behavior*, **45**, 68–80.

Link, B. G., Cullen, F. T., Struening, E., Shrout, P. E. and Dohrenwend, B. P. (1989). A modified labelling theory approach to mental disorders: an empirical assessment. *American Sociological Review*, **54**, 400–423.

Link, B. G., Struening, E. L., Rahav, M., Phelan, J. C. and Nuttbrock, L. (1997). On stigma and its consequences: evidence from a longitudinal study of men with dual diagnosis of mental illness and substance abuse. *Journal of Health and Social Behavior*, **38**, 177–90.

Link, B. G., Phelan, J. C., Bresnahan, M., *et al.* (1999). Public's conception of mental illness, labels, causes, dangerousness and social distance. *American Journal of Public Health*, **89**, 1328–33.

Lipton, F. R., Cohen, C., Fischer, E. and Katz, S. E. (1981). Schizophrenia: a network crisis. *Schizophrenia Bulletin*, **7**, 144–51.

Macias, C., Barriera, P., Alden, M. and Boyd, J. (2001). The ICCD benchmarks for clubhouses: a practical approach to quality improvement in psychiatric rehabilitation. *Psychiatric Services*, **52**, 207–13.

Maclean, U. (1969). Community attitudes to mental illness in Edinburgh. *British Journal of Preventive and Social Medicine*, **23**, 45–52.

Mallett, R., Leff, J., Bhugra, D., Pang, D. and Zhao, J. H. (2002). Social environment, ethnicity and schizophrenia: a case control study. *Social Psychiatry and Psychiatric Epidemiology*, **37**, 329–35.

Mandiberg J. (1995). Can interdependent mutual support function as an alternative to hospitalization? The Santa Clara County Clustered Apartment Project. In *Alternatives to the Hospital for Acute Psychiatric Treatment*, ed. R. Warner. Washington, DC: American Psychiatric Press, pp. 193–210.

Mandiberg, J. M. (1999). The sword of reform has two sharp edges: normalcy, normalization, and the destruction of the social group. *New Directions for Mental Health Services*, **83**, 31–44.

Mandiberg, J. M. (2000). Strategic technology transfer in the human services: a case study of the mental health clubhouse movement and the international diffusion of the clubhouse model. Unpublished Ph. D. thesis. Department of Organizational Theory, University of Michigan, East Lansing, MI.

Manning, C. and White, P. D. (1995). Attitudes of employers to the mentally ill. *Psychiatric Bulletin*, **19**, 541–3.

Marder, S. (1996). Management of treatment-resistant patients with schizophrenia. *Journal of Clinical Psychiatry*, **57** (Suppl. 11), 26–30.

Marshall, J. R. and Funch, D. P. (1979). Mental illness and the economy: a critique and partial replication. *Journal of Health and Social Behavior*, **20**, 282–9.

Mattson, M. R. and Sacks, M. H. (1983). Seclusion: uses and complications. *American Journal of Psychiatry*, **135**, 1210–13.

McCrone, P. and Thornicroft, G. (1997). Credit where credit's due. *Community Care*, **September**, 18–24.

McFarlane, W. R., Dushay, R. A., Deakins, S. M., *et al.* (2000). Employment outcomes in family-aided assertive community treatment. *American Journal of Orthopsychiatry*, **70**, 203–14.

McGuire, T. G. (1991). Measuring the costs of schizophrenia. *Schizophrenia Bulletin*, **17**, 375–8.

McGurk, S. R. and Mueser, K. T. (2003). Cognitive functioning and employment in severe mental illness. *Journal of Nervous and Mental Disease*, **191**, 789–98.

McHugo, G. J., Drake, R. E. and Becker, D. R. (1998). The durability of supported employment effects. *Psychiatric Rehabilitation Journal*, **22**, 55–61.

Meise, U., Sulzenbacher, H., Kemmler, G. and De Col, C. (2001). A school programme against stigmatization of schizophrenia in Austria. Presented at Together Against Stigma, 2–5 September, Leipzig.

Miller, F. E. (1996). Grief therapy for relatives of persons with serious mental illness. *Psychiatric Services*, **47**, 633–7.

Mind (1996). *Not Just Sticks and Stones: A Survey of the Stigma, Taboos and Discrimination Experienced by People with Mental Health Problems*. London: Mind.

Mind (1999). *Creating Accepting Communities: Report of the Mind Enquiry into Social Exclusion and Mental Health Problems*. London: Mind.

Moffit, R. (1990). The econometrics of kinked budget constraints. *Journal of Economic Perspectives*, **4**, 119–39.

Moore, E., Ball, R. A. and Kuipers, E. (1992). Staff–patient relationships in the care of the long-term adult mentally-ill: a content analysis of expressed emotion interviews. *Social Psychiatry and Psychiatric Epidemiology*, **27**, 28–34.

Morgan, R. (1979). Conversations with chronic schizophrenic patients. *British Journal of Psychiatry*, **134**, 187–94.

Morgan, K. (2003). Insight and psychosis: an investigation of social, psychological and biological factors. Unpublished Ph. D. thesis. London: King's College London.

Moscarelli, M., Rupp, A. and Sartorius, N. (1996). *Handbook of Mental Health Economics and Health Policy: Schizophrenia*. Chichester: John Wiley & Sons.

Mosher, L. R. and Burti, L. (1989). *Community Mental Health: Principles and Practice*. New York: W.W. Norton.

Mueser, K. T., Becker, D. R., Torrey, W. C., *et al.* (1997a). Work and nonvocational domains of functioning in persons with severe mental illness: a longitudinal analysis. *Journal of Nervous and Mental Disease*, **185**, 419–26.

Mueser, K. T., Drake, R. E. and Bond, G. R. (1997b). Recent advances in psychiatric rehabilitation for patients with severe mental illness. *Harvard Review of Psychiatry*, **5**, 123–37.

Mueser, K. T., Clark, R. E., Haines, M., *et al.* (2004). The Hartford study of supported employment for persons with severe mental illness. *Journal of Consulting and Clinical Psychology*, **72**, 479–90.

Myers, J. K. and Bean, L. L. (1968). *A Decade Later: A Follow-up of Social Class and Mental Illness*. New York: John Wiley & Sons.

Noble, J. H. (1998). Policy reform dilemmas in promoting employment of persons with severe mental illness. *Psychiatric Services*, **49**, 775–81.

Noble, J. H., Honberg, R. S., Hall, L. L., *et al.* (1997). *A Legacy of Failure: The Inability of the Federal-State Vocational Rehabilitation System to Serve People with Severe Mental Illnesses*. Arlington, VA: National Alliance for the Mentally Ill.

Norman, R. M. G. and Malla, A. K. (1983). Adolescents' attitudes towards mental illness: relationships between components and sex differences. *Social Psychiatry*, **18**, 45–50.

O'Driscoll, C., Wills, W., Leff, J. and Margolius, O. (1993). The TAPS project 10: the long-stay populations of Friern and Claybury Hospitals: the baseline survey. *British Journal of Psychiatry*, **162** (Suppl. 19), 30–35.

Office of National Statistics (1995). *Labour Force Survey*. London: Office of National Statistics.

Office of National Statistics (1998). *Labour Force Survey (1997/8)*. London: Office of National Statistics.

Parker, J. J. (1979). Community mental health center admissions and the business cycle: a longitudinal study. Unpublished Ph. D. thesis. Department of Sociology, University of Colorado, Boulder, CO.

Paykel, E. S., Hart, D. and Priest, R. G. (1998). Changes in public attitudes to depression during the Defeat Depression Campaign. *British Journal of Psychiatry*, **173**, 519–22.

Penn, D. L., Guynan, K. and Daily, T. (1994). Dispelling the stigma of schizophrenia: What sort of information is best? *Schizophrenia Bulletin*, **20**, 567–75.

Phelan, J. C., Bromet, E. J. and Link, B. G. (1998). Psychiatric illness and family stigma. *Schizophrenia Bulletin*, **24**, 115–26.

Polak, P. and Warner, R. (1996). The economic life of seriously mentally ill people in the community. *Psychiatric Services*, **47**, 270–74.

Polak, P. R., Kirby, M. W. and Deitchman, W. S. (1976). Treating acutely ill psychiatric patients in private homes. In *Alternatives to the Hospital for Acute Psychiatric Treatment*, ed. R. Warner. Washington, DC: American Psychiatric Press, pp. 213–23.

Powell, R., Hollander, D. and Tobinasky, R. (1995). Crisis in admission beds. *British Journal of Psychiatry*, **167**, 765–9.

Rabkin, J. (1974). Public attitudes towards mental illness: a review of the literature. *Schizophrenia Bulletin*, **10**, 9–33.

Rabkin, J. G., Muhlin, G. and Cohen, P. W. (1984). What the neighbours think: community attitudes toward local psychiatric facilities. *Community Mental Health Journal*, **20**, 304–12.

Reda, S. (1995). Attitudes towards community mental health care of residents in north London. *Psychiatric Bulletin*, **19**, 1–3.

Reda, S. (1996). Public perceptions of former psychiatric patients in England. *Psychiatric Services*, **47**, 1253–5.

Rees, W. D. (1971). The hallucinations of widowhood. *British Medical Journal*, **iv**, 37–41.

Repper, J., Sayce, L., Strong, S., Willmot, J. and Haines, M. (1997). *Tall Stories from the Backyard: A Survey of "Nimby" Opposition to Mental Health Facilities Experienced by Key Service Providers in England and Wales*. London: Mind.

Rinaldi, M., McNeil, K., Firn, M., *et al.* (2004). What are the benefits of evidence-based supported employment for patients with first-episode psychosis? *Psychiatric Bulletin*, **28**, 281–4.

Roberts, J. D. and Ward, I. M. (1987). *Commensurate Wage Determination for Service Contracts*. Columbus, OH: Ohio Industries for the Handicapped.

Rogers, E. M. (1995). *Diffusion of Innovations*. New York: Free Press.

Rogers, E. M. (1996). The field of health communication today: an up-to-date report. *Journal of Health Communication*, **1**, 15–23.

Romme, M. and Escher, S. (2000). *Making Sense of Voices: The Mental Health Professional's Guide to Working With Voice Hearers*. London: Mind.

Roosevelt, T. (1903). Labor Day speech in Syracuse, New York. Quoted in Andrews, R., Biggs, M., Seidel, M., *et al.* (1996). *The Columbia World of Quotations*. New York: Columbia University Press.

Rosenfield, S. (1992). Factors contributing to the subjective quality of life of the chronic mentally ill. *Journal of Health and Social Behavior*, **33**, 299–315.

Roth, P. (1997). A conversation with Primo Levi by Philip Roth. In *Survival in Auschwitz*, ed. P. Levi. New York: Simon & Schuster/Touchstone, pp. 175–87.

Salyers, M. P., Becker, D. R., Drake, R. E., *et al.* (2004). Ten-year follow-up of clients in a supported employment program. *Psychiatric Services*, **55**, 302–8.

Sartorius, N. (1997). Fighting schizophrenia and its stigma: a new World Psychiatric Association educational programme. *British Journal of Psychiatry*, **170**, 297.

Sartorius, N., Fleischhacker, W. W., Gjerris, A., *et al.* (2002). The usefulness of the 2nd-generation antipsychotic medications. *Current Opinion in Psychiatry*, **15** (Suppl. 1), S7–16.

Savio, M. and Righetti, A. (1993). Cooperatives as a social enterprise in Italy: a place for social integration. *Acta Psychiatrica Scandinavica*, **88**, 238–42.

Scheff, T (1966). *Being Mentally Ill: A Sociological Theory*. Chicago IL: Aldine.

Scheper-Hughes, N. and Lovell, A. M. (1987). *Psychiatry Inside Out: Selected Writings of Franco Basaglia*. New York: Columbia University Press.

Schwartz, G. and Higgins, G. (1999). *Marienthal: The Social Firms Network*. Redhill, Surrey: Netherne Printing Services and Social Firms UK.

Sengupta, A., Drake, R. E. and McHugo, G. J. (1998). The relationship between substance use disorder and vocational functioning among persons with severe mental illness. *Psychiatric Rehabilitation Journal*, **22**, 41–5.

Senn, V., Kendal, R. and Trieman, N. (1997). The TAPS project 38: level of training and its availability to carers within group homes in a London district. *Social Psychiatry and Psychiatric Epidemiology*, **32**, 317–22.

Sensky, T., Turkington, D., Kingdon, D., *et al.* (2000). A randomised controlled trial of cognitive-behavioural therapy for persistent symptoms in schizophrenia resistant to medication. *Archives of General Psychiatry*, **57**, 165–72.

Sherman, P. S. and Porter, R. (1991). Mental health consumers as case management aides. *Hospital and Community Psychiatry*, **42**, 494–8.

Shibre, T., Negash, A., Kullgren, G., *et al.* (2001). Perception of stigma among family members of individuals with schizophrenia and major affective disorders in rural Ethiopia. *Social Psychiatry and Psychiatric Epidemiology*, **36**, 299–303.

Shimon, S. M., Forman, J. D. (1991). A business solution to a rehabilitation problem. *Psychosocial Rehabilitation Journal*, **14**, 19–22.

Signorelli, N. (1989). The stigma of mental illness on television. *Journal of Broadcasting and Electronic Media*, **33**, 325–31.

Simons, K. (1998). *Home, Work and Inclusion: The Social Policy Implications of Supported Living and Employment for People with Learning Disabilities*. York: York Publishing Services.

Singh, S. P., Burns, T., Amin, S., *et al.* (2004). Acute and transient psychotic disorders: precursors, epidemiology, course and outcome. *British Journal of Psychiatry*, **185**, 452–9.

Smith, A. (2002). *Take a Fresh Look at Print*, 2nd edn. London: International Federation of the Periodical Press.

Snyder, K. S., Wallace, C. J., Moe, K. and Liberman, R. P. (1994). Expressed emotion by residential care staff operators and residents' symptoms and quality of life. *Hospital and Community Psychiatry*, **45**, 1141–3.

Sontag, S. (1988). *Aids and Its Metaphors*. London: Penguin.

Star, S. A. (1955). *The Public's Idea About Mental Illness*. Chicago, IL: National Opinion Research Center.

Starks, R. D., Zahniser, J. H., Maas, D. and McGuirk, F. (2000). The Denver approach to rehabilitation services. *Psychiatric Rehabilitation Journal*, **24**, 59–64.

Stastny, P., Gelman, R. and Mayo, H. (1992). The European experience with social firms in the rehabilitation of persons with psychiatric disabilities. Unpublished report. Albert Einstein College of Medicine, New York.

Stroul, B. A. (1988). Residential crisis services: a review. *Hospital and Community Pyschiatry*, **39**, 1095–9.

Stuart, H. and Arboleda-Florez, J. (2000). Community attitudes toward people with schizophrenia. *Canadian Journal of Psychiatry*, **46**, 245–52.

Sturt, E. and Wykes, T. (1986). The Social Behaviour Schedule: a validity and reliability study. *British Journal of Psychiatry*, **148**, 1–11.

Sullivan, G., Wells, K. W. and Leake, B. (1991). Quality of life of seriously mentally ill persons in Mississippi. *Hospital and Community Psychiatry*, **7**, 752–5.

Sullivan, G., Burnam, A. and Koegel, P. (2000). Pathways to homelessness among the mentally ill. *Social Psychiatry and Psychiatric Epidemiology*, **35**, 444–50.

Tait, L., Birchwood, M. and Trower, P. (2004). Adapting to the challenge of psychosis: personal resilience and the use of sealing-over (avoidant) coping strategies. *British Journal of Psychiatry*, **185**, 410–15.

Tarrier, N., Vaughn, C., Lader, M. N. and Leff, J. P. (1979). Bodily reactions to people and events in schizophrenics. *Archives of General Psychiatry*, **36**, 311–15.

Tarrier, N., Barrowclough, C., Vaughn, C., *et al.* (1988). The community management of schizophrenia: a controlled trial of a behavioural intervention with families to reduce relapse. *British Journal of Psychiatry*, **153**, 532–42.

Tarrier, N., Beckett, R., Harwood, S., *et al.* (1993). A trial of two cognitive-behavioural methods of treating drug-resistant residual psychotic symptoms in schizophrenic patients: 1. Outcome. *British Journal of Psychiatry*, **162**, 524–32.

Tarrier, N., Yusupoff, L., Kinney, C., *et al.* (1998). Randomised controlled trial of intensive cognitive behaviour therapy for patients with chronic schizophrenia. *British Medical Journal*, **317**, 303–17.

Taylor, M. S. and Dear, M. J. (1981). Scaling community attitudes towards the mentally ill. *Schizophrenia Bulletin*, **7**, 225–40.

Taylor, P. and Gunn, J. (1999). Homicides by people with a mental illness: myth and reality. *British Journal of Psychiatry*, **174**, 9–14.

Telintelo, S., Kuhlman, T. L. and Winget, C. (1983). A study of the use of restraint in a psychiatric emergency room. *Hospital and Community Psychiatry*, **34**, 164–5.

Thara, R. and Srinivasan, T. N. (2000). How stigmatising is schizophrenia in India? *International Journal of Social Psychiatry*, **46**, 135–41.

Thompson, A. H., Stuart, H., Bland, R. C., *et al.* (2003). Attitudes about schizophrenia from the pilot site of the WPA worldwide campaign against the stigma of schizophrenia. *Social Psychiatry and Psychiatric Epidemiology*, **37**, 475–82.

Thompson, K. N., McGorry, P. D. and Harrigan, S. M. (2003). Recovery style and outcome in first-episode psychosis. *Schizophrenia Research*, **62**, 31–6.

Thornicroft, G. and Rose, D. (2005). Mental health in Europe: editorial. *British Medical Journal*, **330**, 613–14.

Torrey, W. C., Rapp, C. A., Van Tosh, L., *et al.* (2005). Recovery principles and evidence-based practice: essential ingredients of service improvement. *Community Mental Health Journal*, **41**, 91–9.

Tremblay, T., Smith, J., Xie, H. and Drake, R. E. (2004). Impact of specialized benefits counseling services on Social Security Administration Disability beneficiaries in Vermont. *Journal of Rehabilitation*, **70**, 5–11.

Trieman, N. (1997). Residential care for the mentally ill in the community. In *Care in the Community: Illusion or Reality?*, ed. J. Leff. Chichester: John Wiley & Sons, pp. 51–67.

Trieman, N. and Leff, J. (1996). The TAPS project 24: difficult to place patients in a psychiatric hospital closure programme. *Psychological Medicine*, **26**, 765–74.

Trieman, N., Hughes, J. and Leff, J. (1998a). The TAPS project 42: the last to leave hospital – a profile of residual long-stay populations and plans for their resettlement. *Acta Psychiatrica Scandinavica*, **98**, 354–9.

Trieman, N., Smith, H., Kendal, R. and Leff, J. (1998b). The TAPS project 41: Homes for life? Residential stability five years after hospital discharge. *Community Mental Health Journal*, **34**, 407–17.

Trieman, N., Leff, J. and Glover, G. (1999). Outcome of long-stay psychiatric patients resettled in the community: prospective cohort study. *British Medical Journal,* **319**, 13–16.

Turton, N. (2001). Welfare benefits and work disincentives. *Journal of Mental Health,* **10**, 285–300.

US General Accounting Office (1993). Evidence for Federal Program's Effectiveness is Mixed. GAO/PEMD-93–19. Washington, DC: US Government Printing Office.

Valmaggia, L. R., van der Gaag, M., Tarrier, N., Pijnenborg, M. and Sloof, C. J. (2005). Cognitive-behavioural therapy for refractory symptoms of schizophrenia resistant to atypical antipsychotic medication. *British Journal of Psychiatry,* **186**, 324–30.

Van Os, J., Hanssen, M., Bijl, R. V., *et al.* (2000). Strauss (1969) revisited: a psychosis continuum in the general population? *Schizophrenia Research,* **45**, 11–20.

Vaughn, C. and Leff, J. P. (1976). The measurement of expressed emotion in families of psychiatric patients. *British Journal of Social and Clinical Psychology,* **15**, 157–65.

Wagner, L. C. and King, M. (2005). Existential needs of people with psychotic disorders in Pôrto Alegre, Brazil (2005). *British Journal of Psychiatry,* **186**, 141–5.

Wahl, O. (1995). *Media Madness: Public Images of Mental Illness.* New Brunswick, N J: Rutgers University Press.

Wahl, O. (1999). Mental health consumers' experience of stigma. *Schizophrenia Bulletin,* **25**, 467–78.

Warner, R. (2004). *Recovery from Schizophrenia.* Hove and Philadelphia, PA: Brunner-Routledge.

Warner, R. and Polak, P. (1995). The economic advancement of the mentally ill in the community: economic opportunities. *Community Mental Health Journal,* **31**, 381–96.

Warner, R. and Wollesen, C. (1995). Cedar House: a non-coercive hospital alternative in Boulder, Colorado. In *Alternatives to Hospital for Acute Psychiatric Treatment,* ed. R. Warner. Washington, DC: American Psychiatric Press, pp. 3–17.

Warner, R., Taylor, D., Powers, M. and Hyman, J. (1989). Acceptance of the mental illness label by psychotic patients: effects on functioning. *American Journal of Orthopsychiatry,* **59**, 398–409.

Warner, R., Taylor, D., Wright, J., *et al.* (1994). Substance use among the mentally ill: prevalence, reasons for use and effects on illness. *American Journal of Orthopsychiatry,* **64**, 30–39.

Warner, R., de Girolamo, G., Belelli, G., *et al.* (1998). The quality of life of people with schizophrenia in Boulder, Colorado, and Bologna, Italy. *Schizophrenia Bulletin,* **24**, 559–68.

Warner, R., Huxley, P. and Berg, T. (1999). An evaluation of the impact of clubhouse membership on quality of life and treatment utilization. *International Journal of Social Psychiatry,* **45**, 310–21.

Warner, R., Marine, S., Evans, S. and Huxley, P. (2004). The employment and income of people with schizophrenia and other psychotic disorders in a tight labour market. Presented at the WPA International Congress on Treatments in Psychiatry: an Update, 10–13 November, Florence, Italy.

Warr, P. (1987). *Work, Unemployment and Mental Health.* Oxford: Oxford University Press.

Waxler, N. E. (1979). Is outcome for schizophrenia better in nonindustrial societies? The case of Sri Lanka. *Journal of Nervous and Mental Diseases,* **167**, 144–58.

White, T., Ramsay, L. and Morrison, R. (2002). Audit of the forensic psychiatry liaison servison to Glasgow Sheriff Court 1994–1998. *Medicine, Science and the Law*, **42**, 64–70.

Wig, N. N., Menon, D. K., Bedi, H., *et al.* (1987). Expressed emotion and schizophrenia in North India. II. Distribution of expressed emotion components among relatives of schizophrenic patients in Aarhus and Chandigarh. *British Journal of Psychiatry*, **151**, 160–65.

Willetts, L. E. and Leff, J. (1997). Expressed emotion and schizophrenia: the efficacy of a staff training programme. *Journal of Advanced Nursing*, **26**, 1125–33.

Willetts, L. E. and Leff, J. (2003). Improving the knowledge and skills of psychiatric nurses: efficacy of a staff training programme. *Journal of Advanced Nursing*, **42**, 237–43.

Wolff, G., Pathare, S., Craig, T. and Leff, J. (1996a). Community knowledge of mental illness and reaction to mentally ill people. *British Journal of Psychiatry*, **168**, 191–8.

Wolff, G., Pathare, S., Craig, T. and Leff, J. (1996b). Community attitudes to mental illness. *British Journal of Psychiatry*, **168**, 183–90.

Wolff, G., Pathare, S., Craig, T. and Leff, J. (1996c). Public education for community care: a new approach. *British Journal of Psychiatry*, **168**, 441–7.

World Health Organization (1979). *Schizophrenia: An International Follow-up Study*. Chichester: John Wiley & Sons.

World Health Organization (1992). *International Classification of Diseases*, 10th revision. Geneva: World Health Organization.

World Health Organization (2001). *Atlas: Country Profiles on Mental Health Resources 2001*. Geneva: World Health Organization.

Zwerling, I. and Walker, J. F. (1964). An evaluation of the applicability of the day hospital treatment of acutely disturbed patients. *Israel Annals of Psychiatry and Related Disciplines*, **2**, 162–85.

Index

Page numbers in *italics* refer to tables